Field Guide to the Difficult Patient Interview

Field Guide to the Difficult Patient Interview

Frederic W. Platt, MD, FACP, FAAPP
Clinical Professor of Medicine
University of Colorado School of Medicine
Denver, Colorado
Regional Consultant
Bayer Institute for Health Care Communication
West Haven, Connecticut
Staff Physician
Presbyterian/Saint Lukes Hospital
Denver, Colorado

Geoffrey H. Gordon, MD, FACP, FAAPP
Associate Director, Clinical Education and Research
Bayer Institute for Health Care Communication
West Haven, Connecticut
Assistant Clinical Professor of Medicine
Yale University School of Medicine
New Haven, Connecticut
Staff Physician
West Haven Veterans Affairs Medical Center
West Haven, Connecticut

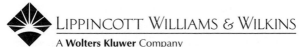
LIPPINCOTT WILLIAMS & WILKINS
A **Wolters Kluwer** Company
Philadelphia · Baltimore · New York · London
Buenos Aires · Hong Kong · Sydney · Tokyo

Editor: Richard Winters
Developmental Editor: Sara Lauber
Marketing Manager: Kathleen Neely
Production Editor: Peter J. Carley
Illustrator: Kim Fraley

351 West Camden Street
Baltimore, Maryland 21201-2436 USA

227 East Washington Square
Philadelphia, PA 19106

Printed in the United States of America

Library of Congress Cataloging-in-Publication Data

Platt, Frederic W.
    Field guide to the difficult patient interview/Frederic W. Platt, Geoffrey H. Gordon.
    p.   cm.
    Includes bibliographical references and index.
    ISBN 0-7817-2044-3
    1. Medical history taking.   2. Physician and patient.   3. Interviewing.
I. Gordon, Geoffrey H.   II. Title. [DNLM: 1. Physician-Patient Relations.
2. C ommunication.   3. Medical History Taking—methods.   W 62
P7189f 1999]
    RC65.P53   1999
    616.07′51—dc21
    DNLM/DLC
    for Library of Congress   99-19265
                                                                    CIP

The publishers have made every effort to trace the copyright holders for borrowed material. If they have inadvertently overlooked any, they will be pleased to make the necessary arrangements at the first opportunity.

To purchase additional copies of this book, call our customer service department at **(800) 638-3030** or fax orders to **(301) 824-7390**. International customers should call **(301) 714-2324**.

99 00 01 02 03
1 2 3 4 5 6 7 8 9 10

DEDICATION

to Brandt Donovan Pepin and Kelsey Emie Pepin

and

to Pat, James, and Colleen Gordon

Preface

From the hundreds of workshops in doctor–patient communication that we have done and from discussions with colleagues throughout the nation, we know that certain encounters are likely to be problematic to both patient and doctor and that it is possible to predict when and why these occur. We know there are procedures and techniques that will help resolve these difficult interactions. By describing those strategies, we intend to help the troubled physician anticipate difficult encounters and recoup quickly when communication between doctor and patient goes awry.

As if dealing with patients weren't difficult enough, doctors now must respond to the needs of numerous oversight organizations, insurance companies, and managed care companies. They all have an interest in improved quality of medical care and better health outcomes, but most physicians and most patients believe that their primary interest is cheaper and faster medicine. We surely have room for improvement in our efficiency, so maybe we can satisfy our own desires for quality while we satisfy some of these organizations' demands for efficiency. The procedures we describe in this book will answer both needs, but only to a point. We have to be able to stand up for what we know is right. If something has to be done and will take time to do, we must take that time.

With all that said, we do know that better communication will improve the mutual satisfaction of doctor and patient in their encounters. We know that better strategies help us avoid disappointment and conflict and increase our efficiency in dealing with patients. We know that improved communication leads to better clinical outcomes for our patients, largely through better agreement between doctor and patient about just what the patient will do. We also know that such communication diminishes the risk of malpractice lawsuits (a happy side effect). Good communication techniques will help us do a more thorough and humane job of doctoring without increasing the time we spend with each patient. By investing time up front in communication that works, physicians can decrease dramatically time spent extricating themselves, their patients, and their patients' families from the morass of misunderstanding, ambivalence, and indirection that defeats so many of our good intentions.

When a new patient comes to our office, we often ask what his goals are and what he hopes to find in a new doctor. The patient usually talks about communication. Just asking such a question opens the door to communication and, more importantly, opens the door to conversing about the *process* of medical interaction.

This book demonstrates how to think about the process of care in order to influence the outcome of care. We believe that communication matters and that communication procedures can be learned. The result of this attention to process by both patient and doctor is a more effective and mutually satisfactory medical encounter.

To achieve efficient and effective communication ourselves, we use a format in this book suggested by Vaughn Keller, Ed.D., at the Bayer Institute for Health Care Communication. Five **P's** guide the reader through complex scenarios and discussions. We introduce a *problem*, describe the *principles* on which an effective approach to the problem rests, offer *procedures* for addressing the problem, list *pitfalls* that threaten the practitioner who aspires to improve, and summarize with the *pearl* at the heart of the chapter.

This short book does not address all the pitfalls and problems in medical interviewing, but we have tried to address the problems that doctors and patients most often mention when asked what frustrates them in their encounters. The skills we demonstrate and recommend, to address the problems listed in the table of contents, are similar to those identified as core communication skills by the American Academy on Physician and Patient. The book is organized in six sections. Part I, "The Efficient Interview," addresses universal techniques that apply both to medical and nonmedical interactions, techniques that will save an enormous amount of time and lead to better results. These techniques have been shown to lead to improvement in five areas: patient satisfaction, physician satisfaction, clinical outcomes, patient adherence to prescribed regimens, and fewer malpractice suits. Part II, "How to Deal With the Difficult Relationship," looks at those heart-sink interactions we all dread and describes techniques and procedures for digging out of such encounters. Part III, "Dealing With Patient Emotions," looks at anger, sadness and fear, grief and ambivalence—dreaded affects that we frequently encounter. Part IV, "Illness and Loss," deals specifically with end-of-life issues, long-term symptoms and suffering, and that medical nemesis, somatization. Part V,

"Behavioral Health Risks," suggests approaches to communication about some key behaviors and health-hazards that our patients bring to us. Finally, Part VI, "Frequent Problems," describes approaches to some difficulties that are growing in frequency as the structure of health care and medical communication changes.

Although the problem encounters we have identified are complex and various, the reader may be comforted to see that for most, we offer a concise group of remedial techniques. They include allowing the patient to tell his or her story uninterrupted, listening in an empathic or reflective way, understanding the differences between acute curable conditions and chronic ones, enlisting the patient as a participant in his or her own care, and practicing self-awareness and self-control. These skills form the basis of every successful interchange, and we believe that mastering them is essential to the happy resolution of any tough encounter.

How should you read this book? We suggest two approaches. You can read it from beginning to end. Or you can read selected chapters when you expect to have, or have just had, a difficult encounter. For example, if you plan an interaction with a patient who has seemed distrustful in the past, read Chapter 10, "Dealing with Distrust of Doctor's Care." If you have just suffered through an encounter with an angry patient, read Chapter 14, "Anger." Either way, we hope you enjoy the book and that it helps you achieve success in these difficult encounters.

Frederic W. Platt, MD
Geoffrey H. Gordon, MD

Foreword

In many respects, this book reflects the coming of age of education in physician–patient communication. Long considered part of the "art" of medicine, physicians' abilities to connect with their patients were considered innate. It was certainly possible to improve one's abilities to communicate through experience, or by emulating a mentor; but as recent as twenty-five years ago, much of the literature on communicating with patients was sparse and anecdotal. Many medical schools at that time simply gave students a list of questions to ask patients on their first clinical rotation.

That has all changed dramatically. George Engel began writing about the medical interview as a core clinical skill and about the need to teach interviewing by observation and feedback. Bird, Cohen-Cole, and Mance developed the "Three-Function Model" of medical interviewing, describing the various skills and subskills of gathering data, building rapport, and giving information. Many wrote books and described curricular innovations to enable students to master basic communication skills. A cadre of researchers proved that enhanced communication skills lead to improved diagnoses, better understanding of patients, enhanced patient satisfaction and compliance, and better health outcomes. Students of Dr. Engel founded the American Academy on Physician and Patient (AAPP), and began faculty development activities that have trained over two thousand teachers of medical interviewing in medical schools and residency programs. The recent AAPP textbook, "The Medical Interview," edited by Lipkin, Lazare, and Putnam, summarizes the many advances in the field. The Bayer Institute of Health Care Communication has trained over 20,000 practicing physicians in effective communication techniques. All these achievements have created an environment in which physician–patient communication is more highly valued and better taught.

Still, there are a number of forces holding back progress in education and practice. The biomedical model is alive and well in U.S. medical education, and many teachers and practitioners are more concerned with patients' diseases than with patients' suffering. The main focus of medical education is on curing diseases (using appropriate drugs or surgery) rather than healing illnesses (which requires the appropriate words, manner, and personal responses to patients' emotions). Medical education, with its rigorous scheduling and often harried attending and house staff, often works against acquiring optimal communication skills. Attending physicians and residents rarely teach or reinforce specific communication strategies on rounds. They more often focus on the interesting "case," on differential diagnosis, on pathophysiology, and on the "numbers." Moreover, the demands of the growing managed care environment leave physicians with less time to focus on their patients' psychosocial concerns. Many physicians who used to be good role models for their trainees are now rushing through patient encounters. Unfortunately, medical education has not responded adequately to the challenges of training physicians for the new realities of practice. Despite better constructed basic communication courses in the preclinical years, medical schools rarely teach and assess students' abilities in the more advanced and subtle skills of communicating with patients in difficult clinical situations. More and more, students are finding that they need to learn these skills by trial and error.

This book is one of the few "field manuals" guiding clinicians through difficult territory in physician–patient communication. The basic skills of eliciting a history, listening actively, expressing empathy, giving information, and offering reassurance are important foundations for students confronting the many challenges in patient care. It also helps to have thought about and mastered the variety of advanced skills and strategies presented in this book before encountering troublesome situations. Also, because one's attitudes, values, biases, emotional reactions, and personal history always affect communication with patients, it can be helpful to reflect on that process. Self-awareness can inform and improve one's abilities to communicate with patients and is the engine for personal and professional growth as a clinician. This growth enables physicians to better use themselves and their emotional reactions to patients for their patients' benefit. This book challenges readers to examine themselves as instruments of diagnosis and therapy and to "calibrate their instruments" through self-awareness. By focusing on basic and advanced communication skills and on personal and professional growth, trainees can realize the ideal of becoming physician-healers.

Fred Platt and Geoff Gordon are remarkably thoughtful and able physicians who have learned much from and have contributed much to the current ferment in the field of physician–patient communication. They have also learned much from their patients and share their collective wisdom in this marvelous book.

Dennis H. Novack, MD
Professor of Medicine
Associate Dean of Medical Education
MCP Hahnemann School of Medicine
Philadelphia, Pennsylvania

Acknowledgments

This book owes its origin to the encouragement of Richard Winters at Lippincott Williams & Wilkins. The book's format stems from suggestions by Vaughn Keller at the Bayer Institute for Health Care Communication and by Sara Lauber and Richard Winters at Lippincott Williams & Wilkins. We are grateful for the editorial help of Constance Platt and Sara Lauber. Constance Platt edited the first three drafts of the book and taught its two doctor–authors to speak English instead of Medicalese. Sara Lauber edited the last two drafts. If the book is readable, it is due to these two superb editors.

The list of topics discussed in this handbook comes primarily from the American Academy on Physician and Patient and the Bayer Institute for Health Care Communication. Both of these organizations have been teaching communication skills to physicians for over a decade. We have been privileged to participate and teach in many communication workshops for these two organizations, and have learned much from the physicians and students who have participated in them. Practicing doctors, residents, and students have told us what communication syndromes trouble them. The American Academy has provided a thoughtful list of advanced medical interviewing skills. The Bayer Institute has provided conceptual models and suggested specific skills.

The ideas in the handbook come from many thoughtful people working in the field of medical communication. The Selected Reading lists appended to each chapter note some of the studies that have most influenced us.

We want to recognize the difficulties of conjoint authorship. As physicians we two have had different kinds of practices. As writers we have different values, different perspectives, and different paces. Working together has given us ample opportunity to practice patience, respect, and the ability to hear, understand and consider the other's viewpoints and ideas. These are the very attitudes we recommend to clinicians working with patients. Over and over in this book, we describe the therapeutic and diagnostic value of reflective listening and empathy. To write a book together required a sizable dose of both. In the end, we two have gained from the endeavor—we've had a lot of fun and both of us have become better physicians through the writing. We hope that it similarly benefits our readers.

Frederic W. Platt
Geoffrey H. Gordon

Contents

Part V: Behavioral Health Risks

Part VI: Frequent Problems

Part I
The Efficient Interview

Part 1

An Efficient Interview

Basic Interviewing Technique

PROBLEM

Doctors and patients alike complain that we don't have enough time together to do our work well. Surely there will never be as much time as we'd like, but we could be more efficient in our work with patients. We need to work smarter.

If we want to be more efficient and effective, we need to engage our patients and enlist them in following our recommendations. The techniques we describe in this first chapter reappear in many different instances throughout this book. They are the bedrock skills of personal and professional communication.

PRINCIPLES

1. Effective communication does not prolong time spent with patients.

2. Communication consists of a set of skills and techniques that can be learned and that will save time once we master them.

3. Paradoxically, we may have to spend more time during the first part of our patient encounters to save time in the long run.

4. Investing time early in building the doctor–patient relationship reduces the likelihood of wasting time later.

PROCEDURES

1. **Begin by attending to the setting.** Identify the people in the room. Exchange names and use them in the subsequent conversation. Sit down, choosing a seat where you can reach the patient; establish eye contact; and be free from intervening obstacles, televisions, or other distractions. Ask your patient if he/she is comfortable and what level of privacy the patient needs to talk freely.

2. **Identify the person of the patient.** Because effective communication is grounded in an understanding of the patient's personal world and not in the abstract clinical details of his/her health, begin your interview with one question in mind: WHO IS THIS PERSON?

When asked how they begin a clinical interview, doctors' responses fall into three groups. About 25% use small talk. "Did you have any trouble getting here with all this snow?" "I see you live in Denver. Are you a Bronco fan?" "Some traffic this morning, eh?" Some 70% tell us that they prefer to "get right down to business," and getting down to business means asking how the patient is feeling: "So what brought you in to see me today?" "What sort of troubles have you been having?" Only a few doctors say they like to begin by asking for personal information. However, there are good reasons to do this, and such an approach usually works smoothly. **Most of your patients will gladly tell you in a few sentences what they consider most important for you to know.** A few will wonder what to say, and you can help them by offering a brief menu:

Dr.: Before we get into the medical stuff, I'd like you to tell me a little about yourself as a person.

Pt.: What do you mean, Doctor?

Dr.: Oh, where you live, who's important in your life, what sort of work you do, what fills your time, you know—whatever is most important for me to understand about you.

Devoting a bit of time to this social history, perhaps a full minute at the onset of the interview, will cement the connection between you and your patient. Knowing the patient as a person will give you a perspective from which to understand the patient's problems. The very act of seeking to know the patient as a person creates a bond that will increase the patient's cooperation with your diagnostic and therapeutic efforts, saving time you would otherwise use trying to convince him/her to follow your recommendations.

In subsequent medical encounters with the patient you can continue to connect at the personal level, demonstrating that, in addition to his/her organs and diseases, you're still interested in how the patient is doing as a person.

3.   **Clarify the patient's agenda.** Early in the interview, try to obtain a complete list of the patient's concerns and desires. **Very few patients come to the doctor with just one problem.** They may be motivated to make the appointment because one issue "drove them to it," but that issue comes with all sorts of auxiliaries. After your initial personal inquiry, begin your investigation: "Before we get too far along, I'd like to know what you'd like to get accomplished here today. What are the problems you're here to talk about?" The patient will begin and want to talk about his/her first problem (often not the most bothersome or worrisome one). You may have to stop him/her: "I see, 'pain

in your knees,' and what's number two on your agenda?" You'll know you've gotten to the bottom of the patient's list when he/she has said "nothing more" at least twice in answer to your "What else?" Only then, when you have a list of problems often too long to handle in that one visit, are you ready to begin your usual interview by asking **which** of all these problems is most troublesome, seeking the chief complaint.

Then you may need to negotiate a consensual agenda, especially if you and your patient disagree over the importance of some of the issues.

> **Dr.:** Well, Mr. A., I see that you have six items on your list. I'm most concerned about the third one, the chest pain. I hear you saying that the ones that especially trouble you are the rash, the diarrhea, and the sore knee. We may not be able to do justice to all these problems today. I want to make sure we address the chest pain today. Which problem is most important to you?

Helping the patient to express all his/her concerns will help you avoid the frustrating "By the way, Doctor" syndrome. That syndrome expresses itself in the patient who saves his/her most important concern or symptom until you think you are finished and are almost out of the room. "By the way, Doctor, what do you do for someone who vomits up blood?"

"By the way ..." is a sure sign that you did not elicit the patient's complete agenda, and hence cannot be sure that you have identified the chief complaint.

4. **Describe the process by which you work.** If you provide a map and signposts, patients are more likely to follow you. Many of our patients are new to the sort of medical care we provide. They may never before have experienced a complete physical examination. They may not understand that one doctor can take major responsibility for much of their health care or that you have to come to a diagnosis before you can attempt effective treatment, so you have to tell them.

> **Dr.:** OK, Mrs. S., I think I understand what brought you here now. What I have to do next is a careful examination and then we have to talk about what might be causing this trouble and what we can do about it. Do you have any questions at this point?   *continued*

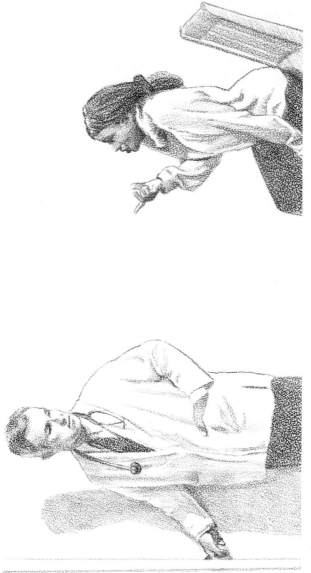

"Oh, by the way, doctor..."

Pt.: An examination? Can't you just prescribe something for the pain and the cough?

Dr.: I wish it were that simple. But I need more information to be sure of the diagnosis, and only then can I make sensible suggestions about therapy. That's why we do an examination.

Pt.: OK, I guess that does make sense. Otherwise you would just have been able to treat me over the phone like Dr. Bell used to do.

Your office staff or the health plan can help your patients to get ready for the visit by instructing them ahead of time how to prepare. They can suggest that patients write down questions and concerns, list the drugs they are taking, and be prepared to answer the doctor's questions about their symptoms. For each problem, most patients have a symptom, a request, and a question and can prepare these ahead of time. The patient can be told ahead of time how long a typical visit will last and can plan how to present his/her agenda. The more prepared your patient is at the beginning of the interview, the more likely he/she is to follow your recommendations at the end.

5. **Consider the patient's narrative.** Part of effective doctoring rests on being able to hear and interpret the story of the patient's illness **as he/she tells it.**

    Mischler's analysis of a series of clinical interactions revealed that doctor and patient seem to be speaking two different languages (Mishler EG. The Discourse of Medicine, 1984). The doctor's language includes the 15,000 new words he/she learns in medical training and is shaped by a world view developed through training in the scientific method. The patient's language is usually a narrative or story that may or may not be chronological. The narrative may be dominated by characters or dramatic incidents and express values that seem to the doctor to be irrelevant to the story of the illness.
    While most patients want to tell stories of their illnesses, most doctors want to hear a synopsis of the medical facts. This conflict between doctors' and patients' discourse goes on all the time.

Dr.: Tell me about this chest pain you're having.

Pt.: Well, first of all you have to understand what happened last year when we were coming back from London.

Dr.: London?

continued

Pt.: Yeah. They had some sort of problem with the airline and they routed us back through San Francisco. It didn't seem so bad, more Frequent Flyer miles and all, but then it was raining in San Francisco and we had three hours to kill. So I walked over to the airport hotel. You know how they have those big cloverleafs there?

There you are, hoping for a few defining parameters of the chest pain, and you get a saga. What's going on? Your patient is telling you about his/her theories of causation, responsibility, and even guilt. You are trying to elicit precise symptoms while you try to fit them into your nascent hypotheses about the potential diseases that might explain the patient's trouble, the unifying diagnosis that Osler spoke about. It seems that you and your patient are speaking two entirely different languages. So what can you do? Mischler says that to communicate effectively you must at least include parts of the patient's story in your bridging request to return to the facts you need.

Dr.: I see. You are concerned that the events of the trip had to do with your pain. But could you first tell me more about the pain itself as it is affecting you now? Where it is, when it happens, what makes it worse or better?

As much as we would like it, we will seldom get "just the facts." We have to hear some part of our patient's narrative if we expect to be successful in our interaction. Even when it does not add to your database, it is therapeutic to your patient to be allowed to tell his/her story. **In fact, the best predictor of patient compliance is the patient's sense of having been heard fully, of having been able to voice all his/her concerns, many of which are not biomedical.**

In the end, doctor and patient have the joint task of constructing a story of the illness that both can agree on. This is not likely to happen if we don't hear the patient's version first. The process of constructing a complete story of the illness resembles a sine wave oscillating between the patient's narrative and the physician's diagnostic reasoning. What doctor and patient are working toward is the creation of a work of art, the history of this illness. Once created, the history will serve as a starting place for all subsequent joint activities. **The process of working together on the history creates a partnership that will help the doctor and patient agree on issues such as who will do what, which later govern the patient's adherence to the medical regimen.**

6. To be an efficient interviewer, strive for precise understanding of the information the patient offers you. You can improve the precision of your understanding by paraphrasing what you have heard and asking the patient to validate the paraphrase. Reiterating what we have heard tells the patient that we are trying to listen and trying to understand. Sullivan compared this iterative process of reflection to following a person through a dark and winding cavern, constantly asking, "Where are you now?" and adjusting your direction on the basis of the response.

This reflection of the biomedical and psychosocial data offered by the patient increases our precision, leading to better diagnosis. **Reflection of our patient's ideas, values, and feelings is the primary tool in empathic communication and is immensely therapeutic to the patient.** Consider these examples of the use of reflection or "short summaries":

i)   Agenda setting:

Pt.: So that's it, doctor. I've got this chest pain, and my knees are aching, and I can't seem to get over the coughing.

Dr.: OK, so if I'm hearing you right, there's chest pain, knee pain, and cough. Anything else?

Pt.: Yeah, one other thing. I haven't been able to have much sex lately. Nothing happens.

Dr.: I see. Pain in chest and knees, cough, and sexual difficulties. What else?

Pt.: That's it, Doc. Isn't that enough?

Dr.: Sounds like enough to me.

---

ii)   Symptom clarification:

Pt.: I had the pain for a week and then this morning I woke up with a crazy rash. I'm broken out, but just over here on the right side where the pain was.

Dr.: So, sounds like you had the pain in your right flank for a week and then today broke out in a rash.

Pt.: Yeah.

---

iii)   Idea validation:

Pt.: I think I've got the gout and I think I need some of that colchicine or something.

Dr.: So what you're telling me is that you think it's the gout and colchicine might be the ticket.

Pt.: Exactly!

iv)   Value validation:

Pt.: The thing is, I really don't want to miss any more work. I've only been on the job a month and I don't want them to think I'm trying to avoid working.

Dr.: I see. It's really important to you that you don't miss any more work.

Pt.: You aren't kidding!

v)   Feeling validation:

Pt.: I don't know, Doc, but I've really been feeling sad since my dog died last month. I know she was old and all that, but she still was always there to greet me when I came home. Now when my wife and I come home, there ain't anyone there to say hello. I really miss the dog.

Dr.: I can understand. You really miss the dog and have been feeling sad since she died.

Pt.: That's it, all right.

Practicing reflective listening or empathy does not add to the total time of the interview. In fact, in our experience it saves time. If the patient does not believe he/she was heard and understood, the patient will repeat the story.

Use care not to overdo it. You need not echo the patient's every symptom, thought, or feeling; but do it periodically to enhance rapport. Above all, try not to miss the most important feelings.

PITFALLS TO AVOID

1.   Ignoring the person of the patient. (After all, we're doctors, not social workers!)

2. Failing to negotiate a consensual agenda for the visit before tackling the first problem the patient offers.

3. Getting impatient when your patient tells a story instead of reciting a list of symptomatic facts.

4. Failing to summarize and reflect what the patient has said, so that you misunderstand the patient and he/she feels ignored or misunderstood.

PEARL

Slow down first to go faster later.

SELECTED READINGS

Beckman HB, Frankel RM. The effect of physician behavior on the collection of data. Ann Intern Med 1984;101:692–96.

Branch WT, Levinson W, Platt FW. Diagnostic interviewing: make the most of your time. Patient Care. July 15, 1996;30(12):68–87

Cassell E. The nature of suffering and the goals of medicine. NY: Oxford Univ Press, 1991.

Delbanco TL. Enriching the doctor–patient relationship by inviting the patient's perspective. Ann Intern Med. 1992;116:414–418.

Engel GL. The need for a new medical model: a challenge for biomedicine. Science 1977;196:129–136.

Greenfield S, Kaplan S, Ware JE. Expanding patient involvement in care: effects on patient outcomes. Ann Intern Med 1985;102: 520–528.

Hall JA, Roter DL, Katz NR. Meta analysis of correlates of provider behavior in medical encounters. Med Care 1988;26:657–75.

Keller VF, Carroll JG. A new model for physician–patient communication. Patient Education and Counseling. 1994;23:131–140.

Korsch BM, Gozzi EK, Francis V. Gaps in doctor–patient communication. 1: Doctor–patient interaction and patient satisfaction. Pediatrics 1968;42:855–71.

Meichenbaum D, Turk DC. Facilitating treatment adherence: a practitioner's guidebook. NY: Plenum Press, 1987.

Mischler EG. The discourse of medicine: dialectics of medical interviews. Norwood, NJ: Ablex Pub., 1984.

Platt FW, Platt CM. Empathy: a miracle or nothing at all. JCOM 1998;5(2):30–33.

Sullivan HS. The collected works of Harry Stack Sullivan. NY: Norton, 1964.

White J, Levinson W, Roter D. Oh by the way, the closing moments of the medical visit. J Gen Intern Med 1994;9:24–28.

CHAPTER 2
Common Problems in Interviewing

PROBLEM

In the ideal interview, the patient presents fact after medical fact, starting with the ones most likely to help us in our search for diagnosis and treatment. The model patient lays before us all the pertinent positive and negative symptoms, unsullied by his/her own ideas of the correct diagnosis; cause of and proper therapy for the problem; or the results of past medical tests, treatments, and doctors' opinions.

In reality, our patients don't know how much we rely on symptoms. They wonder why their current doctor can't just recycle past medical data. Their desire to save time and preserve history is understandable, so we have to explain our need to ask questions that may have been asked before or resign ourselves to continual struggles for control of the interview.

> **Pt.:** So Dr. Berris said that I might have thrombocytopenia and he got a blood count and he said it might be because of an antibody.
>
> **Dr.:** Ms. S., I need to understand better how you've been feeling recently—what sort of symptoms you've been having.
>
> **Pt.:** Symptoms?
>
> **Dr.:** Yes, like pain or shortness of breath or itch or nausea—that sort of thing.
>
> **Pt.:** Oh yeah, I understand what "symptoms" means. I just thought you'd want to know the test results first.
>
> **Dr.:** Well the tests are important, too; but I can help you best if we start with the present, then work backwards to what happened in the past. First tell me how you're not feeling well right now.
>
> **Pt.:** OK. Well, first of all there's this pain in my left side, under my rib cage. Then there's being tired all the time. Then ....

That's where we want to begin.

PRINCIPLES

1. **Only with symptoms can we reach diagnoses.**

2. The cardinal dilemma of interviewing is that we must hear the patient's narrative AND seek a symptomatic history. This dilemma presents itself in almost all of our interviews with patients. Our goal is to get the patient to tell us what we need to hear. Because he/she often tells us what we don't think we need to hear, we are tempted to take over and try to obtain information by a series of questions. Hoping to direct our patient to a symptomatic telling of his/her story, we may overcontrol and end up with the inefficient situation in which we talk more than the patient and our patient answers monosyllabically. The challenge is to put the patient on the right track, then to sit back and let him/her tell us what we need to hear. On the other hand, we have a lot to do, too. We are seeking a clear understanding of the specific details, trying to translate the patient's story into medical data, and forming and testing hypotheses about diagnosis. **The dialectic between our need to understand, sort out, and recombine data and the patient's need to tell his/her story always creates tension in the interview.** We cannot avoid the dilemma; we can only work with it.

3. **As you come to value the patient's narrative more, beware of relaxing your attention to symptoms.** In our experience two sorts of doctors may neglect the need to get a precise account of symptoms: beginners and rapport-builders. The true neophyte, perhaps a beginning medical student, often listens well but settles for a saga of medical care instead of searching for current symptoms. Experienced interviewers who have learned how to use the patient's narrative as a route to better rapport may also fail to get a history rich in symptomatic content. Doctors learning these interview skills may get worse at one part of the interview as they get better at another. Good interviewing rests on maintaining, through minute adjustments, the balance between our patient's narrative and our search for the details we need for diagnosis.

Dr.: Tell me about the trouble you're having.

Pt.: I'm worried about my heart. My Dad died when he was about my age with a heart attack and he was fat like me. So when I started feeling sick, naturally, I thought maybe this was it for me.

Dr.: OK, John, if I understand you correctly, you're concerned about your heart and worried that you may have heart disease like your father did.

continued

Pt.: Right!

Dr.: So now I need you to tell me more about the symptoms that have led you to that concern.

PROCEDURES

1. **Prepare yourself to listen to the patient.**

2. **Be sensitive to the complex internal process you perform as you listen to your patient tell and describe symptoms.** To get all the parameters of the symptoms clarified, you will be listening, reflecting information, and hypothesizing. You will ask clarifying questions. For example, in investigating pain, you want to know where it is first described, where else it is found (radiation), what makes it better (alleviation), what makes it worse (precipitating or aggravating factors), what the time frame is (both short-term for one pain episode and long-term for the overall course of the symptoms), and associated symptoms.

   Our patients will always add descriptors that quantify and qualify their pain. These adjectives and numbers may not be helpful diagnostically, but they increase our understanding of the patient's reaction to the symptom. Meanwhile we must analyze the symptoms and form and test hypotheses, listening intently and then asking clarifying questions. The simultaneity of these activities generates a creative tension in all our interviewing. The fact that we have to do all this while giving the patient room to tell his/her story as the patient sees it; reflecting back what we have heard periodically; and paying close attention to the patient's description of his/her own ideas of causation and of therapy, the patient's values, and his/her feelings; makes interviewing an enormously complex task.

3. **Use "What else?" questions.** To define the parameters for most symptoms, ask **"what else?"** questions to obtain a complete description. By this process of probing, you and your patient will eventually construct a clear history of the illness.

4. Check back with your patient to be sure you got the story right. We suggest checking back periodically with the patient to see that you have understood what he/she is telling you. Where you discover discrepancies, amend your story. Remember that your patient is the source of the historical data. You are the historian.

PITFALLS TO AVOID

1. Forgetting that symptoms are the *sine qua non* of diagnosis.

2. Missing symptoms because you appreciate the importance of hearing your patient's story, including his/her story of tests and results.

3. Wrenching symptoms from the patient by using a highly controlling style, offending him/her with your arrogance.

4. Using questions to test your diagnostic hypotheses before getting the full symptomatic history.

5. Starting to look for symptoms before inquiring about other issues important to the patient, such as what he/she was hoping to accomplish during the visit.

PEARL

Getting the full history of symptoms *efficiently* means sharing control with the patient.

SELECTED READINGS

Burack RC, Carpenter RR. The predictive value of the presenting complaint. J Fam Practice. 1983;16:749–54.

Kaplan C. Hypothesis testing. In: Lipkin M, Putnam SM, Lazare A, eds. The medical interview: clinical care, education and research. Springer-Verlag: NY, 1995;2:20–31.

Kleinman A. The illness narratives: suffering, healing and the human condition. NY: Basic Books, 1988.

Kleinman A, Eisenerg L, Good B. Culture, illness and care: clinical lessons from anthropologic and cross-cultural research. Ann Intern Med 1978;88:251–8.

Mischler EG. The discourse of medicine: dialectics of medical interviews. Norwood, NJ: Ablex Pub, 1984.

Molde S, Baker D. Explaining primary care visits. Image: the Journal of Nursing Scholarship. 1985;17:72–76.

Nardone DA, Johnson GK, Faryna A, Coulehan JL, Parrino TA. A model for the diagnostic medical interview: nonverbal, verbal, and cognitive assessments. J Gen Intern Med 1992;7:437–442.

CHAPTER 3
Patient Education

PROBLEM

Doctors have to explain and educate constantly. The very word ***doctor*** means to lead and to teach. We have to teach about prevention, health maintenance, diagnosis, and treatment.

In order to do this, we have to use a systematic approach to patient education: find out what the patient already knows, ask what the patient wants to know, and talk in terms that the patient understands.

PRINCIPLES

1. We can simultaneously show respect for our patients and simplify the job of educating them by finding out what they already know about the problem before beginning our explanations. More of our educational failures come from not understanding where our patient is than from failing to tell the patient what we think he/she ought to know.

2. Where matters of health are concerned, few of us are dispassionate. To give information successfully to most patients, you will need to understand what feelings are attached to the patient's information about his/her illness.

> **Dr.:** So, John, as you think about this situation, what concerns you the most?

You can use words like "fears" or "worries," but for some patients the less emasculating term "concerns" may get a faster and more forthright response. Some patients, especially male patients, believe that to admit fears is to be cowardly.

> **Dr.:** So, John, as you think about this situation, what are your biggest fears?
>
> **Pt.:** Oh, I'm not really afraid of anything, Doctor. But I did have a couple of questions.

3. The greater variety of communication devices you use, the more likely you are to succeed in explaining. **Use nontechnical words whenever possible. Explain technical terms. Draw pictures.**

Use models, videotapes, and audiotapes. Offer handouts and
articles. Point to key places.

> **Dr.:** John, there are three main arteries that bring blood to the
> muscle of the heart. The heart complains with pain like you
> have if it doesn't get enough blood. But the three arteries aren't
> equally important and their branches are less important. The
> good news is that this one, the left main anterior artery looks
> great. The bad news is that this little branch here seems partly
> plugged up.
>
> **Pt.:** I see. So what do we have to do?

Of course you have to **avoid talking down to your patient.**
You can go too far in simplifying and seeking ordinary nontechnical language. That last explanation might be too simple, even
demeaning, to a cardiac physiologist; but you can excuse over-
explaining ahead of time.

> **Dr.:** John, even though I know that you know more about car-
> diac physiology than I do, I'm going to try to talk with you first
> as if you were an ordinary patient.

4.   You can talk with patients more effectively if you have an idea
     of their most common concerns. Most patients' questions fall
     into two categories: **a) information about health and disease
     and b) concerns about the process of the medical care itself.**
     Questions in the first category are about diagnosis, cause, and
     prognosis. In the second category are questions about what we
     are proposing, how we arrived at those recommendations, what
     the likely outcomes of our proposals might be, and what the haz-
     ards are. If we are doing tests, they want to know when and how
     they will know the results. They also want to know what costs
     they will incur.

5.   **Practicing good medicine means informing the patient.** The
     laws regulating informed consent demand that we tell our pa-
     tients much of what they are eager to hear: what is going on,
     what is likely to occur, what we are proposing to do, and what
     the likely outcomes of our actions might be. We are asked to tell
     our patients about small hazards that occur frequently and about
     large hazards that occur much less often. Patients also want to
     know about the costs they will incur in money, pain, time, and
     risk.

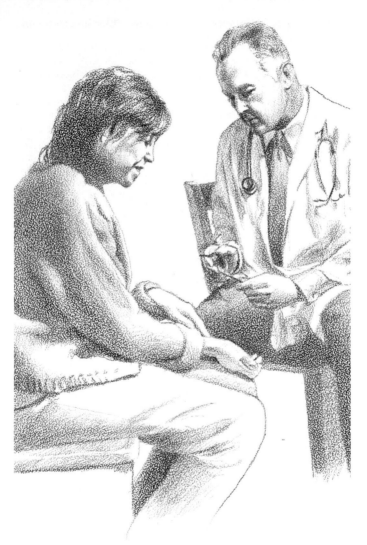

"The more I listen, the more my patients understand."

PROCEDURES

1. Approach your role as educator purposefully, aware that there are certain answers most patients will want and certain information you are required to discuss. **Before addressing your own agenda, ask your patient what he/she thinks is going on, what he/she thinks caused it, what he/she has already tried for it, and what he/she is most concerned about.**

> **Dr.:** John, before we begin, I would like to know what you know about this problem of Hyberk-Schutterfield Syndrome. Tell me how you understand it and what most puzzles you about it.

2. **Ask your patient what information he/she wants from you.**

3. When educating about illness or injury, keep in mind the following checklist. The most common patient questions are:
    a) What is wrong with me?
    b) How did it happen to me?
    c) What is likely to happen next?
    d) What is it you are proposing to do with me and why?
    e) What is the likely outcome?
    f) What should I be worried about? What are the side effects?
    g) If you are doing tests, how and when will I find out the results?

4. **Once you have explained and your patient says that he/she understands, ask the patient to repeat the explanation so you can check to see that he/she understood.** One way of asking for this feedback is to pose a hypothetical case: "When you go home your wife (husband, spouse, significant other) will ask you to tell her what I said, so tell me what you will tell her." Or you can take the role of the person whose explanation might not be clear: "I'd like to be sure I explained myself clearly. Would you please tell me what you heard so that I can see if I've made myself clear?" Although this scenario may take a few minutes, it's time well spent because the patient leaves with information to share, not vague impressions about the illness that have to be clarified in phone calls with worried relatives in the middle of the night.

PITFALLS TO AVOID

1. Assuming that your patient has a good understanding of biological and medical terms and functions.

19

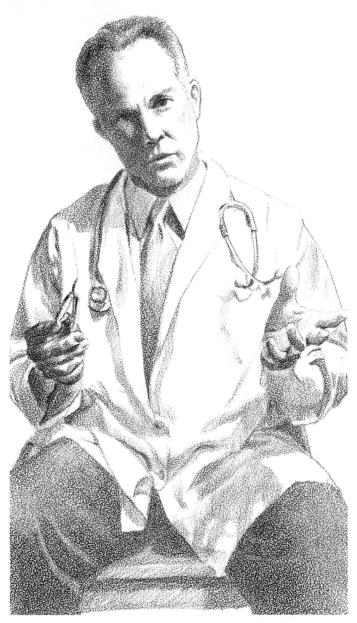

"Let me explain."

2. Failing to find out your patient's ideas and worries about his/her illness.

3. Overlooking important information when educating your patient.

4. Failing to document your explanation in the chart.

PEARL

Tell the patient what he/she wants to know before explaining what you think he/she needs to know.

SELECTED READINGS

Bartlett EE, Grayson M, Barker R, Levine DM, Golden A, Libber S. The effects of physician communication skills on patient satisfaction, recall and adherence. J Chronic Dis 1984;37:755–764.

Calkins DR, Davis RB, Reiley P, Phillips RS, Pineo KL, Delbanco TL, Iezzioni LI. Patient–physician communication at hospital discharge and patients' understanding of the post discharge treatment plan. *Arch Intern Med* 1997;157:1026–1030.

Cassell E. Talking with patients. vol. 1. The theory of doctor–patient communication. Cambridge, MA: MIT Press, 1998.

Cohen JJ. Remembering the real questions. Ann Intern Med 1998;128:563–566.

Falvo D, Tippy P. Communicating information to patients: patient satisfaction and adherence associated with resident skill *J Fam Practice* 1988;26:643–647.

Gordon GH, Duffy FD. Educating and enlisting patients. JCOM 1998;5(4):45–50.

Grueninger UJ, Duffy FD, Goldstein MG. Patient education in the medical encounter: how to facilitate learning, behavior change and coping. In: Lipkin M, Putnam SM, Lazare A, eds. The medical interview. clinical care, education and research. NY: Springer-Verlag, 1995:122–133.

Keller VF, Carroll JG. A new model for physician–patient communication. Patient Educ Couns 1994;23:131–140.

Quill TE, Brady H. Physician recommendations and patient autonomy: finding a balance between physician power and patient choice. Ann Intern Med 1996;125:763–769.

Simpson MA, Buchman R, Stewart M, Maguire P, Lipkin M, Novack D. Doctor–patient communication: the Toronto consensus. BMJ 1991;303:1385–1387.

Waitzkin H. Doctor–patient communication. Clinical implications of social scientific research. JAMA 1984;252:2441–2446.

CHAPTER 4
Translation

PROBLEM

Every clinical encounter is in fact a cross-cultural event. Every conversation between two people involves two languages.

Consider what happens when the patient does not speak your language, nor you the patient's. If he/she comes with a family member to translate, you might experience something like this:

> **Dr.:** Are you having pain?
>
> **Daughter:** Mamacita, el quiere saber si te duele algo.
>
> **Pt.:** Si, tengo muchos problemas con mareos, y mis brazos que no sirven, y con el pecho y mis nalgas.
>
> **Daughter:** She says, "no."

Or, consider this patient who speaks your language but has a different use for the words and a different idea about pathophysiology:

> **Pt.:** I've been having cardiovascular symptoms with my arms. They get numb and feel dead and as if there was a vibrator inside. Then, after I had the chelation therapy I started to get respiratory failure.

PRINCIPLES

1. Disparities in understanding abound, even when we seem to speak the same language.

2. Translators should translate words, meanings, and feelings. Family members seldom make the best translators, but we can help them to be more useful to us by asking them to report a complete version of what the patient said. This may compensate for relatives' desire to edit out culturally embarrassing items.

3. We have to watch out for the **Two Patients Syndrome.** The translator who is a family member may have opinions or feelings about the relative's well-being that distort his/her rendition of the interview. That translator may require your therapeutic attention as well.

4. Even when he/she speaks your language, your patient's ideas about health and illness may be unfamiliar. The patient may report diagnostic and technical terms that do not mean to him/her what they mean to you. He/she may expect a different process of care than you are planning.

5. Many recent immigrants may have medical sophistication far beyond what you'd expect from their current employment.

6. Family involvement is often more than you'd expect. Family members and their ideas may strongly influence the patient's acceptance of your ideas.

PROCEDURES

1. **Learn a second language.** If you live in an area where a large number of your patients speak Spanish as their primary language and you plan to care for them, at least learn medical terms and descriptors in Spanish.

2. **Tell translators what you need to obtain good information.** Set goals, roles, and expectations with your translator. There is a dilemma: you need the translator to do just that, without additions or subtractions. But you also need to allow the translator to pick and explore psychosocial cues and sensitive topics and to help you understand culture-specific beliefs and concerns.

> **Dr.:** Ms. A? I need you to help me communicate with your mother. Can you translate for me? Here's what I need you to do. I need you to sit behind your mother here and to tell her exactly what I say, only in Spanish. Then I need you to tell me exactly what she says, only in English. Don't leave anything out. OK?
>
> **Daughter:** Sure. I can do that.
>
> **Dr.:** OK. But it's hard. I know you know a lot about your mother and will be tempted to add what you know at times. However, what I need first is for you to translate exactly, back and forth.
>
> **Daughter:** OK, I'll try to do that.
>
> **Dr.:** Good. Then, if she says something I wouldn't understand without more explanation, tell me about that too. I'd really like to hear about her concerns. If she says something I wouldn't understand without more explanation, tell me about that too.

3. When the identified patient is accompanied by a friend or rela-
    tive who is doing all the talking, you may have two patients at
    once. Attend to the most distressed person first. Sometimes this
    is not the identified patient, but the one making the most clamor.
    You may have to hear both people.

4. Be sure to elicit your patient's theories of illness causation and
    ideas of treatment, and consider them.

5. Do not use as a translator a family member you suspect of having
    perpetrated abuse or violence against the patient.

PITFALLS TO AVOID

1. Not investing energy in learning a second language, believing
    that English is good enough to convey all you need to know.

2. Assuming the designated interpreter knows his/her job well.

3. Missing the two-patient syndrome.

4. Missing your patient's explanatory model, especially if he/she
    seems to speak your language.

5. Making assumptions about a person's level of medical sophisti-
    cation because of a foreign accent or a less-sophisticated occupa-
    tion.

PEARL

Remember that translation includes culture as well as language.

SELECTED READINGS

Anderson JM, Waxler-Morrison N, Richardson E, Herbert C, Murphy
    M. Delivering culturally sensitive health care. in Waxler-Morrison
    N, Anderson JM, Richardson E, eds. Cross cultural caring: a hand-
    book for health professionals. Vancouver, BC: UBC Press, 1990.
Chuchkes E, Christ G. Cross-cultural issues in patients' education. Pa-
    tient Education and Counseling 1996;27:13–21.
DelBanco TL. Enriching the doctor–patient relationship by inviting the
    patient's perspective. Ann Intern Med 1992;116:414–418.
Hardt E. The bilingual interview and medical interpretation. In: Lipkin
    M, Putnam SM, Lazare A, eds. *The medical interview:* clinical care,
    education and research. NY: Springer-Verlag, 1995;14:172–177.

Martin A. Exploring patient beliefs: steps to enhancing physician–patient interaction. Arch Intern Med 1983;143:1773–1775.

Putsch RW. Cross-cultural communication: the special case of interpreters in health care. JAMA 1988;254:2244–2248.

Welch M, Feldman MD. Cross-cultural communication. In: Feldman MD, Christensen JF, eds. Behavioral medicine in primary care. Stamford CT: Appleton and Lange, 1997:97–108.

CHAPTER 5

Understanding Nonverbal Communication

PROBLEM

What we say nonverbally will always be heard louder than what we say with words. Even when we are trying hard to communicate with our patients, even when we listen carefully and try to use empathic communication, our body language and nonverbal communication may subvert us. To test this assertion, try asking a friend to tell you about something he/she is quite interested in, then turn away and start fiddling with your shoelaces. Your friend will stumble to a halt, be puzzled, but generally conclude that you really don't want to hear from him/her at all.

PRINCIPLES

1. **Your nonverbal language should match the content and intent of your verbal language.**

2. **If your body language says something different than your words, you need to consider what you really want to say.**

3. **Your patient's body language also tells a great deal.** Pay attention to it. If the patient is looking away, maybe he/she doesn't want to hear what you have to say. If the patient has his/her arms folded across the chest, maybe he/she hates hearing what you are saying and is not going to cooperate.

4. **People more often convey feelings and attitudes nonverbally rather than verbally, especially via posture, facial expression, and tone.** Paralanguage—tone, volume, and pace of speech— convey more emotion than words themselves.

    Don't be like one widely admired clinician, who used to make rounds at the hospital with his car keys in his hand. The message to his patients was, "I don't really want to be here. I'm out of here as soon as I can be." Nothing he said convinced his patients that he was interested in their problems.

PROCEDURES

1. **Avoid outside interruptions** when you're with a patient. If you have a secretary or a receptionist, be sure that he/she screens

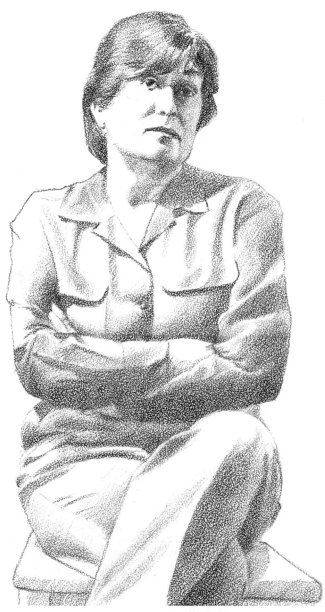

"I'm not listening."

your phone calls and beeper messages. Coach your phone screener how to take messages so that the short-stopping really works.

Secretary: Hello, I'm responding to your page for Dr. X. I'm his assistant, Ms. K.

Dr. Y: Yeah, I need to talk to Dr. X.

Sec.: Dr. Y., Dr. X. asked that he not be interrupted except for emergencies while he's with this patient. Can I have him call you back in 20 minutes? Can you tell me where and how he can best reach you?

Dr. Y.: Well, 20 minutes won't do. He'll have to call me later.

Sec.: OK, tell me exactly when and where I should have him call you.

Without precise answers to these questions, you will either be interrupted or due for a long game of telephone tag with your colleague.

Consider how you prioritize your time with the patient. Studies of house staff time utilization show that they spend less than 20% of their actual time with patients. Yet that time is valued most by the patients and is, indeed, most important to our work. If you value your time with the patient highly, perhaps you can get a colleague to cover for pager and phone calls while you are with the patient. Then you can reciprocate. Interruptions of patient visits are countertherapeutic, and you can ask for help in avoiding them.

2. **Attend to details that make you and the patient more comfortable, like adequate light and privacy.** Don't let charts, computers, tables, or desks come between you and your patient.

3. **Look like you are listening. Sit down.** Establish eye contact, lean forward, focus on what your patient says. Above all, don't talk while you're listening.

4. **Look like you're there for a while**, not just flitting through. **Sit down**, sitting close enough so you can touch your patient at appropriate times. Try to sit at eye level with the patient. (Some emergency departments have bought captains' stools so doctors can sit at the same level as a patient on an elevated gurney.)

5. **Use touch appropriately.** Some patients distrust touch, others avidly seek it. Try to be alert to your patient's responses to touch.

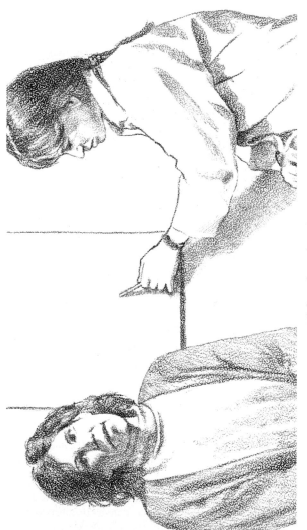

High-tech explanation

A patient who smiles and speaks more vigorously when his/her hand is touched is different from one who flinches. Most patients, describing painful or fearful or sad moments, appreciate a gentle touch on wrist or elbow, an I'm-here-with-you gesture. If you begin your interview with a handshake, generally a good idea, you have already initiated touch and can more naturally reach out again as "touching" parts of the conversation occur.

PITFALLS TO AVOID

1. Not bothering to sit down, since you won't be there long. Standing over your patient.

2. Staring at the chart or computer instead of attending to the patient.

3. Taking pages or phone calls during the interview. Popping in and out of the room will impress your patient with how hard you work and how important you are, although not with how much you value his/her visit.

PEARL

Even when you're not talking, your body language is talking for you.

SELECTED READINGS

Baldwin JG Jr. The healing touch. *Am J Med* 1986;80:1.

Bruhn JG. The Doctor's Touch: tactile communication in the doctor–patient relationship. *South Medical J* 1978;71:1469–1473.

Darwin C. The expression of the emotions in man and animals. 3rd edit. NY: Oxford Univ Press, 1998.

Di Matteo MR, Taranta A, Friedman HS, Prince LM. Predicting patient satisfaction from physicians' nonverbal skills. Med Care. 1980;18(4):376–387.

Drasselhaus TR, Luck J, Wright BC, Spragg RG, Lee ML, Bozzette SA. Analyzing the time and value of house staff inpatient work. J Gen Intern Med 1998;13:534–540.

Giron M, Manjon-Arce P, Puerto-Barber J, Sanchez-Garcia E, Gomez-Beneyto M. Clinical interview skills and identification of emotional disorders in primary care. *Am J Psychiatry* 1998;155:530–535.

Hall JA, Roter DL, Rand CS. Communication of affect between patient and physician. *J Health Soc Behav* 1981;22:18–30.

Larsen KM, Smith CK. Assessment of nonverbal communication in the physician–patient interview. *J Fam Pract* 1981;12:481–488.

Oddone E, Guarisco S, Simel D. Comparison of housestaff's estimates of their workday activities with the results of random work-sampling study. Acad Med 1993;68(11):859–861.

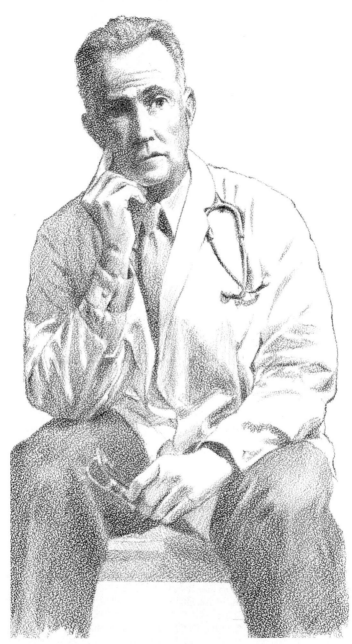

"I'm here to listen."

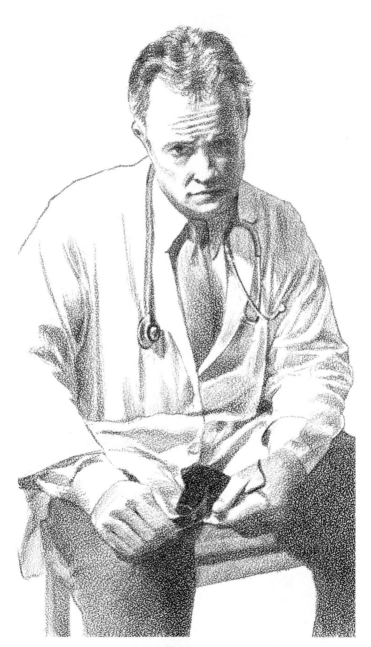

Concern

Rowland-Morin P, Carroll JG. Verbal communication skills and patient satisfaction: a study of doctor–patient interviews. *Eval and Health Prof* 1990;13:168–185.

Silverman J, Kurtz S, Draper J. Nonverbal communication. In: Skills for communicating with patients. Oxford: Radcliffe Medical Press, 1998:73–79.

CHAPTER 6
Listening

PROBLEM

Patients say that they want their doctors to listen to them and to understand them. This is not a surprising request. It's something we all want. But do we have the time to listen? Do we even know how? **Inaccurate and ineffective listening leads to diagnostic and therapeutic disasters and convinces our patients that they are in the hands of incompetents.** Consider these two examples. In the first case, the doctor was forewarned that he was to admit a patient with chronic obstructive lung disease, thus his interest in the possibility of dyspnea:

> **Dr.:** OK, Mr. A., what sort of trouble have you been having?
>
> **Pt.:** Well, I've had some trouble with my legs and ....
>
> **Dr.:** (interrupting) Have you had trouble breathing?
>
> **Pt.:** Well yes, I always have some trouble with my breathing. See I have emphysema and ....
>
> **Dr.:** (interrupting) Are you coughing? Coughing anything up?
>
> **Pt.:** No, not really. It's just that ....
>
> **Dr.:** (interrupting) So is there chest pain?
>
> **Pt.:** No. No chest pain.
>
> **Dr.:** What medicines are you taking?

Later, this doctor said that taking a history from Mr. A. was like pulling teeth. The patient said that this doctor was arrogant and didn't listen to him. He then amended his description to, "Dr. X. is probably a good doctor, but you can't talk to him."

In the second case, both Dr. Y. and Dr. Z. interviewed Mr. B. at different times. Neither checked back with the patient to see if they had heard him correctly. Both were eager to get on with their questions. They both believed that the main task of the interview was to get the answers to their questions, and that the best way to do that was to ask all their questions as efficiently as they could. When asked why they selected that form of interviewing, both responded that asking questions saves time.

Here's how Dr. Y. recounted his patient's story:

Dr. Y.: Mr. B. is about 70 and has had gall bladder disease for about three years. His pain attacks are becoming more frequent and he came into the hospital for an elective cholecystectomy.

Here's what Dr. Z. gleaned:

Dr. Z.: Mr. B. is about 65 and he's been having epigastric and substernal pain, especially when he lies down. He gets a little relief from chewing antacid tablets. He's concerned that heart disease is the cause of his trouble.

Here's what Mr. B. said:

Patient B: I'm 72. I used to be a telephone lineman but I'm retired now. I've been pretty healthy and so has my family except that my Dad died when he was 76 with a heart attack. My problem is my gall bladder and I'm going to have to have it out. It hurts here (pointing to epigastrium) and runs up under my breastbone. Used to be a few Tums would solve the pain but now the pain seems more bothersome.

Each interviewer identified a piece of the elephant. Unfortunately, the patient's surgeon heard only the first piece of information and, convinced that the patient was suffering from gallstones, removed an asymptomatic gall bladder. The patient's esophageal pain continued.

Fortunately there are ways to become more efficient and more effective listeners.

PRINCIPLES

1. **Listening requires being quiet and paying attention to the person who's talking.** When you listen, you note the content of what you've heard. Many of us spend the time when another person is talking planning for what we will say next. That's not listening. At the very least, allow your patient to finish his/her opening statement. In one study, the average doctor's interruption of the patient came only 18 seconds into the interview. Once interrupted, patients never finished their opening statements. If uninterrupted, the average opening statement lasted less than 90 seconds, much shorter than many of us expect.

2. **Only the patient's validation can confirm your understanding of his/her story.**

3. **The inquiry through which you elicit medical data from the patient is not an inquisition.** The interview is a dance in which you and the patient should alternate leading.

4. **Look for symptoms.** Your patient will tell you his/her own diagnosis, theories of causation, and ideas about prognosis and therapy. You must hear and validate these theories while at the same time mining for symptoms—the gold of the interview.

PROCEDURES

1. **To show that you are listening, sit or stand at eye level with the patient.** Whenever possible do your interviews sitting down—it looks more like you are there to stay and shows both interest and patience. You must show these even if they are not what you're feeling.

2. **Listening requires silence on your part. Let the patient talk without interruption.** If you are a sub-eighteen–second interrupter, try spending a full minute listening without interruption. Interruption includes the clarifying questions like "how long?" and "exactly where?" and "what makes it better?" that we all love and that you know you will have to ask sooner or later. Ask these questions a bit later than your instinct dictates. **Use nods, grunts, and other non-verbal facilitation.** Before asking questions that can be answered with a "no," a "yes," or a number, give open directions or ask open-ended questions such as "Go on." or "What else?" or "Then what?"

    Remember that any question that can be answered with a number or a "yes" or a "no" is not an open-ended question.

3. **Summarize the story for your patient and ask for correction, then incorporate the corrections into your next version.** This iterative process should continue throughout the interview. You can even explain it to your patient:

Dr. X.: Mr. C?

Pt.: Yes?

continued

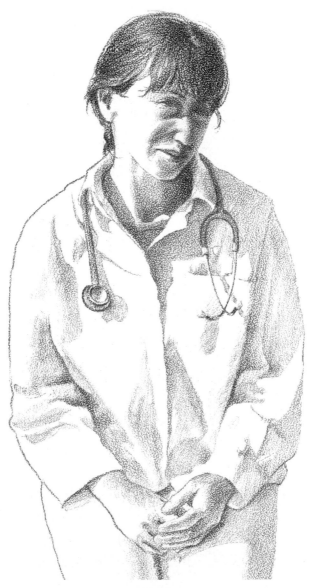

Listening

Dr. X.: I'd like to tell you what I've understood as we go along and get corrections from you. OK?

Pt.: Sure, Doc. OK with me.

4. **Gently insist on the most precise version of any information about symptoms your patient can offer.**

Pt.: So I've had this pain for quite awhile.

Dr.: I see. Quite awhile. How long might that be in days or months or years?

Pt.: Oh, I don't know, Doc, a long time.

Dr.: Mmmm. Like, how long is a long time to you?

Pt.: Oh gosh, maybe six months or so. Maybe a year? I don't know.

Dr.: I understand; you haven't kept exact track of the time. But sounds like about six to twelve months or so.

Pt.: Yeah.

5. **Categorize the data you obtain for yourself and for your patient.**

Pt.: So I've had this trouble with my gall bladder and need to have it out. It gets me right here (points) and sometimes wakes me up and I have to chew up about three tablets before I feel OK and can lie back down.

Dr.: So the **symptoms** are mostly pain under your breastbone and you **think** probably the trouble stems from those gallstones you told me about and that maybe you need to have your gall bladder removed?

Pt.: That's it, Doc. That's why I'm here.

Note the key words? "Symptoms" points to the relevant medical facts, and "think" notes the patient's ideas of diagnosis, causation or correct therapy.

PITFALLS TO AVOID

1. Disrespecting your patient as a potential source of useful information by rushing the patient through his/her story. Interrupting eagerly and often.

2. Ignoring the need to form a working relationship with the patient in order to enlist him/her in subsequent plans.

3. Believing that your chief interviewing task is to get answers to your specific questions and not to tolerate any interruptions.

4. Discounting the possibility of your mishearing or the patient misspeaking. Not checking by reflecting the data and asking for validation.

5. Failing to reflect because you lack key opening words like "Let me see if I have understood you right," or "So it sounds like you are ...."

PEARL

Listen to your patient. Don't get just a piece of the elephant.

SELECTED READINGS

Beckman HB, Frankel RM. The effect of physician behavior on the collection of data. Ann Intern Med 1984:101;692–696.

Frankel RM, Beckman HB. Accuracy of the medical history: a review of current concepts and research. In: Lipkin M, Putnam SM, Lazare A, eds. The medical interview: clinical care, education and research. NY: Springer-Verlag, 1995:511–524.

Platt FW, McMath JC. Clinical hypocompetence: the interview. Ann Intern Med 1979;91;898–902.

Platt FW, Platt CM. Empathy: a miracle or nothing at all. JCOM. 1998;5(2):30–33.

Rowland-Morin PA, Carroll JG. Verbal communication skills and patient satisfaction: a study of doctor–patient interviews. Evaluation and the Health Professions. 1990;13(2):168–185.

Silverman J, Kurtz S, Draper J. Internal summary. In: Skills for communicating with patients. Oxford: Radcliffe Medical Press, 1998:65–69.

Smith RC, Hoppe RB. The patient's story; integrating the patient- and physician-centered approaches to interviewing. Ann Intern Med 1991;115:470–477.

Suchman AL, Markakis K, Beckman HB, Frankel R. A model of empathic communication in the medical interview. JAMA 1997;277: 678–682.

Weisberg J. Does anybody listen? does anybody care? Englewood, CO: Medical Group Management Association, 1984; 27–38.

Part II
How to Deal With the Difficult Relationship

CHAPTER 7
Acknowledging Difficult Relationships

PROBLEM

Physicians tend to blame patients for most of the difficult interactions they experience, and patients blame doctors. Unfortunately, it does little good to blame each other for the trouble. But instead of considering that we ourselves might be causing the trouble or that the problem lies in a troubled relationship, we more often sound like these three doctors.

> **Dr. X.:** What really bugs me is a patient who doesn't respect me, one who reads a magazine in the clinic when I'm trying to talk to him or takes phone calls or watches TV while I'm with him in the hospital room.
>
> **Dr. Y.:** Yeah, and even worse are the patients who want to argue about my diagnosis or who think they know the right therapy before they even consult me.
>
> **Dr. Z.:** I agree. There are a lot of difficult patients out there.

Yes, both patients and doctors can be difficult, but most frequently doctor–patient interactions are difficult. A better approach is to view the relationship as derailed and find an approach to get it back on track.

PRINCIPLES

1. Although either doctor or patient can remedy a dysfunctional interaction, it is usually the doctor who wields the most influence and has the best chance to repair the interaction.

2. Repair work for a disrupted interaction can require considerable thought and attention. All elements of the interaction (the doctor, the patient, the illness, and the environment) can contribute to the difficulty. Interactions may suffer from minor ills (e.g., the patient who is watching television while you are trying to conduct an interview), or major ones (e.g., the patient who disagrees with your diagnosis and your idea of the right treatment).

3. A dysfunctional interaction between the doctor, the patient, the medical disorders, and the environment often occurs when one or both parties perceive success to be unlikely, when their ex-

pectations are misaligned, or when both lack the necessary flexibility.

PROCEDURES

1. **Recognize the difficulty early.** You may be tipped off to the trouble when you notice repetition, interruption, or stereotypic behavior on the part of yourself or the patient. A global sense of distress or a great desire to be somewhere else may be the first signal that the interaction is failing.

2. Once you are aware that something is going wrong, pause, step back, and think about the matter. You and your patient need a time-out, a moment of silence, or a brief separation while you think about the interaction.

> **Dr.:** Mr. Apple, I need to stop for a moment and think about what you have been saying and what's going on.
>
> **Pt.:** And on, and on, and on ....
>
> **Dr.:** No, really, Mr. Apple (touching the patient on his knee), I really need to stop for a minute. Please don't tell me anything else until I think a bit.

3. Acknowledge to yourself that you are having difficulty and probably also some feelings about it. Are you angry? Sad? Feeling trapped? For many of us, these feelings happen so fast that we act on them before thinking. Being aware of your feelings and knowing what they mean can help you identify what went wrong and what needs to be done differently.

4. **Come up with a differential diagnosis for the problem you are experiencing in the interaction.** Be careful. You are not diagnosing your patient's problem (for example a personality problem or lack of social support, even though these may be true). At this point, you are naming a problem in the doctor–patient interaction itself.

5. Check to see if the disruption stems from a strong affect in the patient: anger, sadness, fear, or the feeling of being caught in a bind. If so, address that feeling first, using empathic responses.

6. If the problem has not been caused by a strong patient affect, **try sharing the problem you are facing with your patient**, and ask

him/her for help. Avoid blaming or name-calling. In fact, you may be able to own the entire problem and ask your patient for help.

Dr.: I think we're kind of stuck here, Mr. A., and I think the problem I'm having is that I hear you telling me about a whole lot of separate problems and I don't know where we should start. Can you help me by telling which is giving you the most trouble?

In acknowledging your discomfort, you are asking the patient to be a partner in resolving what seems to be an interactional problem. Sharing the problem may be quite simple and fairly brief. For example, when something in the interview environment becomes a distraction:

Dr.: Wait a second, Mr. B. I've just realized that the television set is on and that sometimes it's distracting me or you. Can we turn it off?

Pt.: Sure, Doc. I'm not in the hospital just to catch up on my soap operas, you know.

Sometimes sharing the problem may require a longer dialogue, with negotiated solutions:

Dr.: Mr. C., the way I see it, we'd be successful if you finished your course of physical therapy, your pain management therapy, and your vocational rehabilitation.

Pt.: I don't see it that way at all. I need compensation for my pain and suffering and, by the way, I'm out of those pain medicines. I need you to refill the prescription and fill out those disability papers.

Dr.: So we have really different ideas about what we think success is.

Pt.: You wouldn't let a dog suffer like this, Doc.

Dr.: I can understand how frustrating it would be to be suffering as you are and then to find that your doctor has ideas that are pretty different from yours. But we do differ on goals.

Pt.: You aren't kidding.

continued

45

Dr.: Do you see any way we can work together?

Pt.: I'll take anything that will get me back on my feet.

Dr.: That sounds like a goal I'd agree with too. So what can we do?

Pt.: Well, if I stay in the therapy and the rehab program, can you keep giving me the pain meds?

Dr.: Yes. I think so.

PITFALLS TO AVOID

1. Blaming the patient for stirring up your own bad feelings.

2. Riding roughshod over troubling interactions.

3. Ignoring the patient's strong affect.

PEARL

Give prompt attention to difficult interactions.

SELECTED READINGS

Carroll JG, Platt FW. Engagement: the grout of the clinical encounter. J Clin Outcomes Management 1998;5(3):43–45.

Gorlan R, Zucker HD. Physicians' reactions to patients: a key to teaching humanistic medicine. N Eng J Med 1983;308:1059–1063.

Kemp-White M, Keller VF. Difficult clinician–patient relationships. J Clin Outcomes Management 1998;5:32–36.

McCue JD. The effects of stress on physicians and their medical practice. N Engl J Med 1982;306:458–463.

Novack DH, Suchman AL, Clark W, Epstein RM, Najberg E, Kaplan C. Calibrating the physician: personal awareness and effective patient care. JAMA 1997;278:502–509.

Platt FW. Acknowledgment. In: Conversation repair: case studies in doctor–patient communication. Boston: Little, Brown, 1995;3: 59–100.

Quill TE. Recognizing and adjusting to barriers in doctor–patient communication. Ann Intern Med 1989;111:51–57.

Quill TE, Williamson PR. Healthy approaches to physician stress. Arch Intern Med 1990;150:1857–1861.

Zinn WM. Doctors have feelings too. JAMA 1988;259:3296–3298.

CHAPTER 8
Understanding the Meaning of Illness

PROBLEM

In clinical medicine, there is always more to discover, especially about how things look to the patient. We do a fairly good job at listing and characterizing symptoms and at diagnostic reasoning. We do less well eliciting and understanding the meaning of the illness as the patient sees it, even though that meaning often drives the patient's behavior.

> **Dr.:** So what we need to do is get you into the hospital and give you some medicines to dry you out. You're choking with all this excess water. We ought to have you better in a day or two.
>
> **Pt.:** Not on your life.
>
> **Dr.:** What?
>
> **Pt.:** I'm not going into the hospital. Nope. If I have to die, I'm going to do it at home.
>
> **Dr.:** Who said you have to die?
>
> **Pt.:** Doesn't matter. I'm not going.

Here's a turn of events we hadn't anticipated. We have to discover more.

PRINCIPLES

1. We are not finished with the medical interview until we discover what the illness means to the patient.

2. We can look for symbolic meaning, functional meaning, and relational meanings of the illness.

3. The route to understanding is to ask the patient to explain what the illness and its therapy mean to him/her.

PROCEDURES

1. Assume that every patient has a unique sense of his/her illness: its cause; its effect on the patient's life; and what needs to happen for him/her to get better.

2. When the patient responds in a way that puzzles us, or that doesn't make sense given what we know and have said, we should assume we're probably missing the meaning of the illness to the patient. Rather than accuse the patient of self-destructiveness or resistance, accept the fact that we have more to discover. We can phrase our response to the patient in this way.

> **Dr.:** Mr. A., I don't yet understand how things look to you.
>
> **Pt.:** Whatever you understand, I'm not going into the hospital.
>
> **Dr.:** OK, I do understand that part—you're not going into the hospital. No matter how it looks to me, you're not going. Right?
>
> **Pt.:** Right!
>
> **Dr.:** OK. But what I'd like to understand better is how this illness and this hospital business look to you. Tell me more about it.
>
> **Pt.:** What do you want to know?

3. **What we want to know includes:**

   a) How the illness and the recommended treatment affect our patient's **roles** as employee, spouse, caregiver, parent, and so on.

   b) How the illness and the recommended treatment affect our patient's **relationships**—family, friends, and work colleagues.

   c) **What concerns the patient has about the illness or the treatments.**

   d) What this illness or treatment symbolizes to the patient. What does the patient **think the illness says about him/her as a person?** e.g. "I should have worn my coat," or "I should have gone to church more," or "I'll never write that novel now." We can ask, "How do you think about yourself differently because of this?"

4. **Don't be afraid to expose your ignorance.** "I still don't understand. Can you help me understand better?" or "I'm curious to know how this looks to you. Can you tell me more?" are questions that show our concern as well as a desire to understand.

> **Dr.:** I can see that you're not going to the hospital. Can you tell me what keeps you from going?
>
> **Pt.:** I can't. My wife will be home alone. She's helpless and depressed. She might kill herself. I can't leave her home alone.

Knowing this, you might be able to start considering how to solve your stand-off with the patient.

PITFALLS TO AVOID

1. Assuming that if things are not going in the direction you would choose, it is because the patient is resistant to your ideas, is in denial as to the seriousness of his/her plight, or is stubborn.

2. Getting into an argument. Repeating your views again, believing that your job is to convince the patient rather than understand the patient.

> **Dr.:** Look, there's no other way about it. You're going into the hospital.
>
> **Pt.:** Oh yeah?

3. Failing to consider other possible therapeutic routes, believing that it's your way or the highway.

PEARL

Try to discover at least three things that the illness means to the patient.

SELECTED READINGS

Barsky III AJ. Hidden reasons some patients visit doctors. Ann Intern Med 1981;94:492–8.

Connelly JE, Campbell C. Patients who refuse treatment in medical offices. Arch Intern Med 1987;147:1829–33.

Connelly JE, Mushlin AI. The reasons patients request "checkups": implication for office practice. J Gen Intern Med 1986;3:164–5.

Delbanco TL. Enriching the doctor–patient relationship by inviting the patient's perspective. Ann Intern Med 1992;116:414–8.

Hilfiker D. *Healing the wounds: a physician looks at his work.* NY: Pantheon, 1985.

Kemp-White M, Keller VF. Difficult clinician-patient relationships. J Clinical Outcomes Management 1998; 5(5): 32–36.

Martin AR. Exploring patient beliefs. Steps to enhancing patient physician interactions. Arch Intern Med 1983;143:1773–5.

Platt FW. Discovering meaning. In: Conversation repair: case studies in doctor–patient communication. Boston: Little, Brown, 1995: 1–22.

CHAPTER 9

Addressing Disagreements About Diagnosis or Therapy

PROBLEM

Much more frequently than we would wish, doctors and patients fail to agree on the diagnosis or the correct course of therapy. When that happens, the patient invariably refuses to follow the doctor's instructions. To make ourselves more effective doctors, we need a technique to address these disagreements.

PRINCIPLES

1. The patient's beliefs and theories about his/her illness—its cause, diagnosis, and prognosis—are important to discover, to recognize openly, and to discuss with your patient because they will affect his/her acceptance of your help and his/her cooperation in it.

2. Working with your patient's theories includes respecting them. The scientific model of understanding the world through hypothesis testing and empiric research is relatively new, compared to other models that are much easier to understand. We may or may not agree on the benefits of prayer, wheat germ, or chakra balance to remedy illness, but we must respect the various beliefs our patients hold. **Your medicine may be only one of the remedies your patient will try.**

3. Empathic communication is the tool to use in discovering the patient's hypotheses about the diagnosis, cause, and treatment of his/her illness. Empathic communication begins with listening, and if the patient does not volunteer hypotheses about his/her illness, you can ask.

4. Disagreements between the doctor's and the patient's version of diagnosis or treatment can be worked out over time. This comes about through a dynamic relationship that respects each person's opinions and flexibility. Here again you demonstrate that you are with the patient for the long haul.

5. **Write down your goals, intentions, and efforts at providing medical care.** In the worst case, if your patient refuses what you consider to be the best medical care, documentation of your conversations may save you from lawsuits later.

PROCEDURES

1. If you discover a major disparity between your theory and that of your patient, try to put the difference on the table so you can both look at it. One physician says that he likes to place the disparity on a lily leaf and gently float it out on the little pond that lies just between him and his patient. We like that gentle metaphor.

Dr.: Hmm. I think I understand what's happening. I think that we have pretty different views of what's going wrong.

Pt.: What do you mean, Doc?

Dr.: Well, if I understand you right, you have been thinking that you probably have sinusitis, an infection in your sinuses.

Pt.: Right!

Dr.: And I, on the other hand, am more concerned about this chest pain you have been having. I'm concerned that you could have pneumonia or even a blood clot in your lung, a pulmonary embolism.

Pt.: I see.

Dr.: So, given this difference of opinion, how are we to proceed?

Pt.: Well, could we try some antibiotics first? If it's my sinuses, wouldn't that clear it up?

Dr.: Might do it. But if it's really a pulmonary embolism and you have another one, that could cause you serious harm or even kill you. That's the worry I have.

---

2. Recognize that **opening up the disagreement for conversation begins the process of negotiation.** In the above case further negotiation would likely lead to a plan first to rule out the most worrisome diagnosis, the pulmonary embolism, then to go back to the patient's diagnosis and try treating it.

3. If the patient insists on a procedure or treatment that you had not thought appropriate, consider it. **Openness to what your patient is saying, whether you agree or not with his/her theory, is an act of respect.** The patient is more likely to accept an alternative hypothesis after seeing that his/her own has been accorded respect. **Try to learn how the patient has come to his/her opinion and what is motivating it.**

Dr.: Let me see, Mr. F. I hear you saying that you think you need a CT scan of your head. I'm still not sure I understand exactly how you made that decision. Can you fill me in?

Pt.: I just need one, doctor. I don't even want to discuss it.

Dr.: I see. So you believe that you need a CT scan, I don't think you do, and I'm not to know why you think you do? That makes it kind of hard on me to figure out any reasonable route. Are you sure you can't give me a few more hints?

Pt.: Oh, OK. It's just that my wife said I wasn't to come home without one. She says that I either have to quit complaining about the headaches or get a CAT scan. One or the other.

Dr.: Oh! So in fact, you're trapped. You either get a CAT scan or face the music at home.

Pt.: That's about it.

Dr.: OK. I would like to propose a third route. What if we tried the medications I want to prescribe for a week or ten days. You could put all the responsibility for that decision on me when you told your wife. Then, if we weren't successful, we could get a CAT scan even though I am quite confident that it will be normal and that we'll still be in the same muddle therapeutically.

Pt.: I could do that, Doc. Yeah.

4. In confronting the differences between you and your patients, practice empathic communication, an effort to understand the other and to let him/her know that you do understand. Notice the two key lines in that last scrap of dialogue?

Dr.: Oh, so in fact, you're trapped ....

Pt.: That's about it.

The doctor expresses an understanding of how the patient might be feeling and the patient completes the interchange by confirming the accuracy of that understanding.

5. Try to stand on the same side of the street as your patient. You can even use that metaphor in your conversation.

> **Dr.:** OK, I see that we have a difference of opinion. I'd like to come over where you are sitting (moves his chair) so I can see how things look from your point of view.
>
> **Pt.:** That's pretty funny, Doc. You moving over here like that. I've never seen a doctor do that before.
>
> **Dr.:** I imagine. Well, now that I'm over here next to you, explain again how it all looks to you, what's wrong and what we ought to do. I may not agree but I sure want to understand your point of view as well as I can.

6. If the negotiation fails, you may be able to agree to disagree. You can end gracefully and part peacefully even if you and the patient have radically different ideas of what should be done.

PITFALLS TO AVOID

1. Getting offended and settling into an intransigent position.

> **Dr.:** Look, I'm the doctor here! What we need to do is treat this with an H-2 blocker for a week or two.
>
> **Pt.:** That stuff never works for me. You need to send me to a gastroenterologist so he can look down there again.
>
> **Dr.:** Oh yeah? Who's in charge here?

  This conversation is stuck with two parties taking fixed positions and neither hearing the other. In a healthy clinical relationship both the doctor and the patient are in charge—a partnership. Here it seems to be one or the other.

2. Repeating yourself, only louder ad infinitum.

> **Dr.:** I don't think it's sinus trouble.
>
> **Pt.:** Well, doctor, I really do think it is.
>
> **Dr.:** No, I don't think it's your sinuses. No, not at all.

3. Failing to understand your patient's ideas or values. Almost surely your patient's decision will reflect a cost—benefit analysis he/she has made, albeit unconsciously, about the issues.

> **Pt.:** You know, Doc, whatever else happens, I want my wife to be satisfied with what we do.
>
> **Dr.:** OK, let's just try the antibiotics first.

4. Missing golden opportunities for empathic communication.

> **Pt.:** My wife says have a CAT scan or don't come home.
>
> **Dr.:** Well, I think we should try the antibiotics first.

PEARL

Ask: What leads your patient to think what he/she thinks?

SELECTED READINGS

Brody DS. The patient's role in clinical decision-making. Ann Intern Med 1980;93:718–722.

Duncan BL. Stepping off the throne. Networker 1997;July:23–33.

Ende J, Kazis L, Ash A, Moskowitz MA. Measuring patients' desire for autonomy: decision making and information-seeking preferences among medical patients. J Gen Intern Med 1989;4:23–30.

Fisher R, Ury W. Getting to yes: negotiating agreement without giving in. Boston: Houghton Mifflin, 1981.

Gross R, Birk PS, D'Lugoff BC. The influence of patient–practitioner agreement on the outcome of care. Am J Public Health. 1981;71: 127–132.

Lazare A. The interview as a clinical negotiation.. In: Lipkin M, Putnam SM, Lazare A, eds. The medical interview: clinical care, education and research. NY: Springer-Verlag, 1995:50–64.

Lazare A, Eisenthal S, Wasserman L. The customer approach to patienthood. Arch Gen Psychiatry. 1975;32:553–8.

Quill TE. Partnerships in patient care, a contractual approach. Ann Intern Med 1983;98:228–234.

Quill TE, Brody H. Physician recommendations and patient autonomy: finding a balance between physician power and patient choice. Ann Intern Med 1996;125:763–769.

Tuckett D, Boulton M, Olson C, Williams A. Meetings between experts. NY: Tavistock Pub, 1986.

CHAPTER 10
Dealing With Distrust of Doctors' Care

PROBLEM

Why should our patients trust us? What does "trust" mean, anyway? Usually we expect people to trust us when we are credible or believable, i.e., if we are telling them the truth and they perceive that. Medical behavior that strengthens trust includes our being dependable and putting the patient's interests first; but we cannot simply assume that being honest with our patients will lead them to trust us. Their trust or distrust of us will be qualified by previous medical and life experiences. Patients' old beliefs based on racial or cultural experiences may corrupt our caring and truth-telling and make it hard for patients to trust us. Some people, patients or relatives, will distrust you because they have never learned to trust anyone; others will distrust you because their picture of what you might offer differs strikingly from what you *can* offer. And some people are convinced that all doctors should be approached with a protective shield of distrust. On the other hand, many of our patients say it behooves them as patients to trust their doctors, a behavior or posture of theirs rather than something we create by our behavior.

Doctors in training often report a special case in which the patient seems doubtful that they really are doctors.

Questions of qualifications come more frequently to younger doctors and female doctors. They are vulnerable to distrust.

> **Pt.:** You say you're my doctor? You look awfully young. Have you taken care of many heart patients before?

PRINCIPLES

1. **Trust is largely a product of good communication.** Patient surveys and focus groups indicate that trust is closely associated with the quality of doctor–patient communication. Malpractice literature shows that patients disenroll from care or bring suit when communication is faulty. Most studies indicate that communication and interpersonal skills are greater determinants of trust than biomedical technical competence.

    Above all, the patient's perception of being treated with respect, being heard, and being understood leads to the phenomenon of trust in the doctor.

2. Just as patients need to trust their doctors, doctors need to be able to trust their patients. If that trust is lost, for example when a doctor learns that his/her patient has been intentionally hiding or distorting important data, the doctor and the patient must discuss the breach of trust and define future limits if the physician is to continue caring for the patient.

3. The more your patients understand medical care, including the uncertainties and imperfections, the more likely they are to trust you—a seeming paradox.

4. Trust should be fair game to discuss openly.

PROCEDURES

1. **Be willing to discuss the patient's or family's distrust.** Watch for opportunities to empathize with the person suffering from distrust.

Dr.: It sounds like you are worried about your mother's health and you are not sure you can trust the very person who is in charge of her care. That makes it pretty tough for you.

Daughter: It's just that I want her to have the best care and I think maybe last time she was in the hospital we should have called in more specialists.

Dr.: I see. You're concerned that we perhaps didn't have enough experts involved. Is there anything else? Anything you're upset with me about that I did or didn't do in the past?

---

2. Try to contain your anger or feelings of distress about not being trusted. Sometimes we become defensive when we think we don't get the trust we deserve. We start to explain all the good things we have done. We may even feel victimized. **Focus on the patient or distrustful party and learn more about him/her.** This is an opportunity to understand more.

Dr.: Lisa, we always talk about your mother and her medical troubles. I wonder if you could tell me how her illness is affecting you? How is it to be trying to care for an elderly and frail mother?

continued

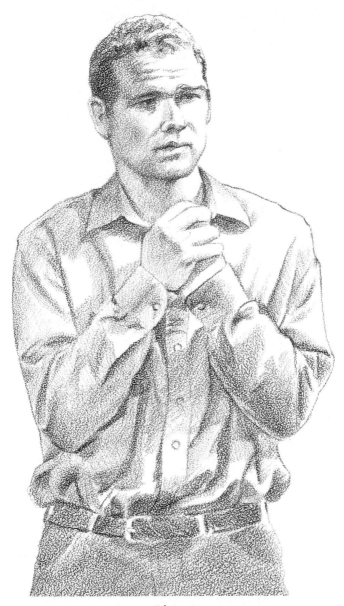

Distrust

Daughter: Sometimes it's not very easy. Everyone seems to depend on me. It's the same at our restaurant. Everything depends on me, and I just can't do everything anymore.

Dr.: I didn't know. Tell me more about that.

This person has a real life with real difficulties and brings those issues to her relationships, including the relationship with her mother's doctor.

3. **Ask what would help the person trust you more.**

Dr.: Lisa, given what you've told me about your mother's illness and how it's been for you, I can understand how you might find it hard to trust me or another doctor. What could I do to help you trust me more?

4. The house staff syndrome can be approached best with understanding.

Dr.: I can imagine that it might be tough for you to find a young, female doctor as part of your health-care team. I'm the doctor writing the orders and notes in your case, but we all discuss it together. My goal is to be sure you get the best medical care from our team. Will that work for you?

PITFALLS TO AVOID

1. Assuming that the patient's lack of trust is really about you. Becoming defensive.

2. Failing to discuss the trust issue, viewing it as too intimate or embarrassing for discussion.

3. Failing to learn more about the distrustful person's life, concerns, values, and thoughts.

PEARL

Don't be afraid to ask about trust.

SELECTED READINGS

Beckman HB, Markakis KM, Suchman AL, Frankel RM. The doctor–patient relationship and malpractice: lessons from plaintiff depositions. Arch Intern Med 1994; 154(12):1365-1370.

Berger JT. Culture and ethnicity in clinical care. Arch Intern Med 1998;158:2085–2089.

Entman SS, Glass CA, Hickson GB, Githens PB, Whetten-Goldstein K, Sloan FA. The relationship between malpractice claims history and subsequent obstetric care. JAMA 1994;272:1588–1591.

Gray BH. Trust and trustworthy care in the managed care era. Health Aff 1997;16(1):31–49.

Johnson GT. Restoring trust between patient and doctor. N Engl J Med 1990;322:195–197.

Kao AC, Green DC, Davis NA, Kaplan JP, Cleary PD. Patients' trust in their physicians: effects of choice, continuity, and payment method. J Gen Intern Med 1998;13:681–686.

Kass NE, Sugarman J, Faden R, Schoch-Spana M. Trust: the fragile foundation of contemporary biomedical research. Hastings Cent Rep 1996;26(5):25–29.

Levinson W, Roter DL, Mullooly JP, Dull VT, Frankel RM. Physician–patient communication: the relationship with malpractice claims among primary care physicians and surgeons. JAMA 1997; 277:553–559.

Mechanic D, Schlesinger M. The impact of managed care on patients' trust in medical care and in their physicians. JAMA 1996;275: 1693–1697.

Miyaji, NT. The power of compassion: truth-telling among American doctors in the care of dying patients. Soc Sci Med 1993;36:249–264.

Newcomer LN. Measures of trust in health care. Health Aff 1997; 16(1):50–51.

Safran DG, Taira DA, Rogers WH, Kosinski M, Ware JE, Tarlov AR. Linking primary care performance to outcomes of care. J Fam Practice 1998;47:213–220.

Thom DH, Campbell B. Patient–physician trust: an exploratory study. J Fam Pract 1997;44:169–176.

CHAPTER 11
Establishing Boundaries

PROBLEM

Although usually unstated, there is a contract between the patient and the doctor with implicit agreement about roles (who will do what), rules of discourse (limits we will observe with each other), and agendas (plans about what to attend to during the visit). When we disagree about roles, rules of discourse, or agendas, the resulting conflicts cripple our interactions.

> **Pt.:** I just need you to sign these disability papers and I'll be out of here.
>
> **Dr.:** Disability papers? Why is that? Who's disabled?
>
> **Pt.:** Me! You know, my back. I can't do my work anymore.
>
> **Dr.:** But I haven't examined your back. You said you were consulting a back expert your company sent you to.
>
> **Pt.:** Yeah, I was. But that ran out. He's done. Now I need you to fill out these forms.

The doctor was distressed by this request because he thought his role as primary physician would include disability claims only if he had examined the patient and had all the information that the other doctor had. He and his patient had different concepts of his role.

Doctors provide many examples of doctor–patient conflict that stem from differing ideas of roles, rules of discourse, and agendas.

Role Disagreements

a) The patient thinks you're responsible for rulings his/her HMO made.

b) The patient thinks you will help him/her receive insurance compensation for a problem that you think you can help the patient overcome.

c) The patient wants you to refill narcotic pain medication endlessly while you want to find another approach to chronic pain.

d) The patient expects you to cure his/her disability, but you think you have to help the patient find ways to live with it.

Differing Ideas About Rules of Discourse

a)   The patient tries to tell his/her story, and the doctor interrupts so
     soon and so often that the patient starts answering with monosyl-
     lables. (The patient's expectation of the conversation is that
     he/she will be allowed to tell his/her story; the doctor's idea is
     that he/she will get answers to his/her questions.)
b)   The patient asks questions but doesn't listen to the answers.
c)   Your new patient wants to call you by your first name on the first
     visit and reaches over and touches you while telling his/her story,
     making you feel uncomfortable.
d)   The patient calls you at home in the evening with a nonemergent
     problem, one that you think should have been dealt with during
     office hours.

Agenda Difference

a)   The patient schedules a fifteen-minute office visit and brings a
     list of ten problems to discuss.
b)   The patient makes an appointment for one child and then brings
     in four, and asks you to examine all of them in the time slot
     you've set aside for one.

PRINCIPLE

To be effective the doctor must acknowledge conflicts and, where possible, negotiate them. The doctor can bring the matter up for discussion
and simply note it as "two differing points of view," then ask the patient about how to proceed.

PROCEDURES

1.   If you are feeling discomfort in the interaction with your patient,
     stop and consider: are boundaries threatened or crossed? Could
     the problem be a matter of disagreement about who does what
     (roles), what you talk about and how you talk about it (rules of
     discourse), or what you can agree on and work together to
     achieve (agenda)?

2.   If so, begin a discussion of the issue.

> **Dr.:** Mr. H., I'm having a little difficulty here and I'd like to
> share it with you.
>
> **Pt.:** Huh? What do you mean, Doctor?
>
> *continued*

Dr.: Well, I think you and I have somewhat different ideas about what I should be able to do for you. I think you believe that I can simply fill out this disability form without examining you.

Pt.: That's it. You got it.

Dr.: Whereas I think my role is to examine you and come to my own conclusion about disability only after I've seen the x-rays, done an examination, and probably conferred with your other consultants. To decide on disability in situations like this I need the opinion of a good neurosurgeon or orthopedist, too.

Pt.: So you're not going to sign the form?

Dr.: Well, not without examining you. But the difficulty seems to me that we have two different points of view about what I ought to do, indeed about what I CAN do. What do you think?

Pt.: Yeah, I guess so. I kind of thought you wouldn't want to just sign the form.

Dr.: So, if we don't just do that, let's talk about how we could proceed and what I COULD do for you. OK?

Pt.: OK, Doc.

3. Most conflicts arise because **two adults have different points of view.** Avoid blame and name-calling:

Dr.: OK, I see.

Pt.: See what, Doc?

Dr.: I see that you are a manipulator. You're trying to sneak this disability form past me. You're trying to pull a fast one on me.

Pt.: I'm what? What gives you the idea you can say that to me? I pay for this medical care you're supposed to be giving me. That's what I pay my insurance for. You doctors are all alike. You don't do a damn thing for anyone and then all you want to do is send your bill and take trips to Europe!

Dr.: Oh yeah? ....

> **The key to effective communication about boundaries is to clarify respect for your patient's and your own boundaries and find ways to discuss them together.**

4. **Avoid thinking of yourself as a victim of the patient with whom you have conflict.**

> **Dr. X.:** WHEN are they going to send someone to me who doesn't have twelve problems on his list and expect me to handle them all in ten minutes?
>
> **Dr. Y.:** WHEN are they going to send someone to me who can answer a simple question with a simple answer instead of a saga?

Drs. X. and Y. aren't victims; they are simply dealing with common problems. Few patients have a clear idea how much time we have or how much time we need to deal with all their problems. All of our patients have stories. We have to hear them.

5. When rules of communication are dramatically broken, such as with disruptive behavior (cursing, demanding, threatening, producing a weapon, hinting at sexual relations ....), **you can respond with a clear statement of limits.**

> **Pt.:** (loudly) You God-damned doctors don't give a shit about patients. All you want is your money.
>
> **Dr.:** Mr. A., I'm uncomfortable when you swear. It makes it impossible for me to do my job as a doctor. Would you like me to step out for a few minutes while you get control of yourself?

Notice that this doctor does not respond in kind; but he does confront the patient squarely about his disruptive behavior, offer a cool-down period, and leave the choice of how things will proceed with the patient.

PITFALLS TO AVOID

1. Getting upset about boundary issues—roles, rules of discourse, and agenda differences —rather than analyzing them.

2.   Failing to involve the patient in solving the dilemma.

3.   Viewing these difficulties as arising outside your interaction, per-
      haps sent to bother and victimize you.

PEARL

Interview difficulties often stem from disagreements about roles, rules
of discourse, and agendas.

SELECTED READINGS

Quill TE. Partnerships in patient care: a contractual approach. Ann In-
      tern Med 1983;98:228–234.
Quill TE, Brody H. Physician recommendations and patient autonomy:
      finding a balance between physician power and patient choice. Ann
      Intern Med 1996;125:763–769.
Quill TE, Suchman AL. Uncertainty and control: learning to live with
      medicine's limitations. Humane Med 1993;9:109–120.
Sparr LF, Rogers JL, Geahrs JO, Mazur DJ. Disruptive medical pa-
      tients: forensically informed decision making. West J Med 1992;
      156:501–506.
Stoudemira A, Thompson TL. The borderline personality in the medi-
      cal setting. Ann Intern Med 1982;96:76–79.
White MK, Keller VF. The difficult clinician–patient relationship. J
      Clin Outcomes Management 1998;5(5):32–36.

CHAPTER 12
Avoiding Seduction

PROBLEM

We and our patients get in trouble when we shift the focus of our interaction from the patient and his/her health needs to some other activity that we both enjoy. This other activity may be sexual, which is the most common interpretation of "seduction." But in most cases where the medical encounter deviates, it involves personal interests shared by doctor and patient: a hobby, a sport, or even the doctor's family. The problem is as much one of a seducible doctor as it is one of a seductive patient.

> **Dr.:** How've you been doing, Audrey?
>
> **Pt.:** Pretty much the same. How about you?
>
> **Dr.:** OK, I guess. Not working too hard this week.
>
> **Pt.:** Doing any writing? Any new poetry?
>
> **Dr.:** Not much. I think I wrote a good one last week though.
>
> **Pt.:** Oh, good! I'd like to see it.

What do you think? Seductive patient? Seducible doctor? This doctor and his patient are poets and have traded their poems back and forth. A pretty platonic relationship, eh? But not necessarily a medical one. Or is it?

> **Dr.:** You know, Audrey, I think we ought to do a little medicine here. Sometimes we get sidetracked from your health and spend all our time talking about literature, especially our own.
>
> **Pt.:** I don't think so, Fred. After all, you keep telling me that a patient's health is as much mental as physical. When we talk about our writing, that's therapeutic for me.

So there's the dilemma. Physicians who have overstepped sexual boundaries sometimes attempt to excuse their behavior the same way: "It was good for the patient." Rarely true; but even if it was, it wasn't medicine. More problematic is the therapeutic property of sharing a common experience or a common interest. Even then, the act of turning to address that interest may move us from our therapeutic focus on the patient.

Some of the tangential attentions that we define as seductions have as their roots the physician's very human needs to be admired, loved, respected, obeyed, or nurtured. Because the physician–patient relationship is so powerful, patients may seek to deepen and intensify it beyond the boundaries of medicine.

PRINCIPLES

1. It is very difficult to know if you have crossed a boundary when you have little sense of where your boundaries in professional relationships lie. **You will benefit from spending some time defining what you believe your boundaries must be in working with patients.** Duckworth and colleagues suggest asking four questions (Duckworth KS, Kahn MW, Gutheil TG, 1994):
    a) Is this what a doctor does?
    b) Do I sense how the patient experiences this?
    c) Is what I am doing for the patient, rather than for me?
    d) Is the healthy side of my patient being supported by my action?

    If the answer to any of these questions is "no," there may be a potential for deprofessionalization of the relationship, for boundary-crossing, or for violation.

2. **The patient is our focus.** We function on a continuum of involvement with our patients. The more we find commonalities, the more we usually like the patient and the more we are tempted to spend time talking about those commonalities. We slip into trouble when we have moved from talking about the patient to talking about ourselves.

3. You can describe the dilemma to your patient. If the patient hopes for more from the relationship, your explanation will be not only clarifying but face-saving.

4. You will develop strong feelings for some of your patients. The work of medicine is often close to love, and caring for the patient, for the very person of the patient, may include great affection. You must be alert to its possible subversion.

5. **Stay alert to the meaning of gifts and invitations.** Often they are simple expressions of gratitude for care. Sometimes, though,

there are strings attached—such as an expectation that special favors (caring, consultations, medications) will ensue.

When reciprocating with special care in response to gifts begins to feel like a burden, it's time to examine the relationship and acknowledge the issue with your patient. At the least, we can assure our patient that he/she will get excellent care with or without the gift. Then we may need to define and set boundaries on what excellent care is.

6. Doctors are experts at delaying gratification, working compulsively, and feeling under-valued. Our work also provides physical and emotional intimacy with our patients. These circumstances make some physicians vulnerable to personal overinvolvement with patients.

PROCEDURES

1. In the interview, **you may digress from health issues but you must come back to them.** Whatever your starting point, try to return to health concerns. "I need to go back and review your health status now."

2. **Stay alert to the problem.** Throughout much of this book we recommend that you view your patient as much more than a biomedical entity, that you come to know who he/she is as a person, that you focus on both psychosocial and biomedical dimensions of the patient. Despite that larger focus, you must retain your role of doctor, not buddy, business partner, or lover. Be aware of this dilemma and you are less likely to get caught in it.

3. **Try to keep the focus of attention on your patient.** Watch for conversations with your patient where YOU have become the focus. That's a clue that you may have been seduced.

4. **No sex, and interpret that rule in its broadest context.** If you and your patient become lovers, your patient will lose a good doctor and gain a mediocre lover. Such a change of roles is illegal, immoral, and foolish. Don't do it.

PITFALLS TO AVOID

1. Forgetting that the lesser seductions like sociability are a greater temptation than acting out erotic love for a patient.

2. Failing to realize that, paradoxically, the better you are at doctoring (i.e., the more you are concerned with the whole patient), the more easily you will be sidetracked from medical issues.

3. Failing to think about temptations like gifts or conjoint family, social, or business activities as potentially destructive to the doctor–patient relationship.

PEARL

Always ask yourself whether the activity you are contemplating with your patient is for your benefit or for the patient's.

SELECTED READINGS

Council on Ethical and Judicial Affairs, American Medical Association. Sexual misconduct in the practice of medicine. JAMA 1991; 266:2741.

Duckworth KS, Kahn MW, Gutheil TG. Roles, quandaries, and remedies: teaching professional boundaries to medical students. *Harv Rev Psychiatry* 1994;1:266–270.

Farber NJ, Novack DH, O'Brien MK. Love, boundaries and the patient–physician relationship. Arch Intern Med 1997;157:2291–2294.

Frankel RM, Williams S. Sexuality and professionalism. In: Feldman MD, Christensen JF, eds. Behavioral medicine in primary care: a practical guide. Norwalk, CT: Appleton and Lange, 1997:30–38.

Gabbard GO, Nadelson C. Professional boundaries in the physician–patient relationship. JAMA 1995;273:1445–1449.

Gutheil T, Gabbard G. The concept of boundaries in clinical practice: theoretical and risk management dimensions. Am J Psychiatry. 1993;150:188–196.

McCue JD. The effects of stress on physicians and their medical practice. N Engl J Med 1982;306:458–463.

C H A P T E R   1 3
Asking for Help

PROBLEM

Sometimes we need to reach outside of the doctor–patient dyad for help. Caring for patients, we are used to asking for help with technical knowledge and procedures. Sometimes we need help to find influence, support, and advocacy for our patients.

PRINCIPLES

1. Help may come from family members, friends, co-workers, other health-care professionals, social service professionals, support groups, or spiritual advisors. Your patient may have a number of helpers of which you are unaware.

2. Helpers should be invited into the doctor–patient relationship to ensure continuity and nonabandonment.

3. The patient should be included in the decision to involve others and be informed of options and consequences of working with others, including how issues of confidentiality will be addressed.

4. Using help requires careful planning, and when the patient is involved you have to allocate responsibility. What will the patient do? What will you do? Who will make key decisions? When a consultant or referral is to be used, that person must understand what your needs are and how communication is to be handled.

5. **It is useful to have an advisor to help determine that you are observing legal reporting requirements**, policies, and system rules. Doctors need help, too.

PROCEDURES

1. Consider carefully what sort of help is needed and where that help might be found. Can the family offer it? Can social agencies? Can the neighbors? Can the church community?

2. **Include the patient in the decision to go outside for help.** Ask your patient what resources he/she wants to use and has available. Is that person available? Is the family to be involved? Does the patient agree with the plan? Is it a plan the patient can work with?

3. **Invite the helpers you call on to join you in the relationship with the patient** for as long as needed, making the arrangement an inclusion of the new helper rather than a sending-away of the patient.

4. **Make sure all parties know who will do what, when it will get done, and how future communications will go.** Be careful to not drop your patient between helpers.

PITFALLS TO AVOID

1. Forgetting to ask your patient whom he/she usually consults in times of need.

2. Trying to solve everything yourself.

3. Losing the patient somewhere between various experts and sub-specialists.

4. Forgetting to tell your consultants what you want and when you no longer need help.

PEARL

Your patient's usual helpers are your best resources.

SELECTED READINGS

Kemp-White M, Kellar VF. Difficult clinician–patient relationships. J Clinical Outcomes Management 1998;5(5):32–36.
Bursztajn H, Barsky AJ. Facilitating patient acceptance of a psychiatric referral. Arch Intern Med 1985;145:73–75.

Part III
Dealing With Patient Emotions

Part III

Dealing With Patient Problems

CHAPTER 14
Anger

PROBLEM

We cannot be effective physicians without addressing patients' feelings as well as their symptoms. The loss of a sense of well-being can stir up strong feelings in people: fear, grief, and anger. If your patient is chronically ill, it's likely that any or all of these feelings lie beneath the surface of your interactions. The most difficult of these feelings is anger.

Nobody likes a confrontation with an angry person; but if we have to endure one, most of us feel we have the right to return the anger if we choose. Doctors, however, don't have that choice when dealing with an angry patient.

Lipp says that doctors who are confronted with an angry person generally employ three techniques, all destined to fail (Lipp. Respectful Treatment, 1986):

a) They disregard the anger, i.e., they keep going, questioning, explaining, acting "normal," and hoping to get past the anger.
b) They try to placate, generally infuriating the angry person and making matters worse.
c) They return anger for anger, a strategy that leads to war.

We have seen a fourth futile response: they attempt premature validation of the patient's anger. This can get you in trouble in two ways. Validation without understanding leads to the patient feeling dismissed. Taking sides, a judgmental stance, teaches the patient to react to your likes and dislikes, which is not always therapeutic.

Strong affect, whether anger, sadness, or fear, unnerves most of us. It's tough enough doing our diagnostic and therapeutic tasks in a calm atmosphere. To maintain the ambiance we need, we must have techniques to move the patient who is in the throes of powerful emotions to a calmer place where we can work together.

PRINCIPLES

1. **Anger, especially anger aimed at you, is an attack and you will feel it as such.** Watch your response and keep it within the bounds that you believe will help rather than make the situation worse.

2. **Empathy is the most effective response to the patient's anger.** We describe empathy as an understanding of values or

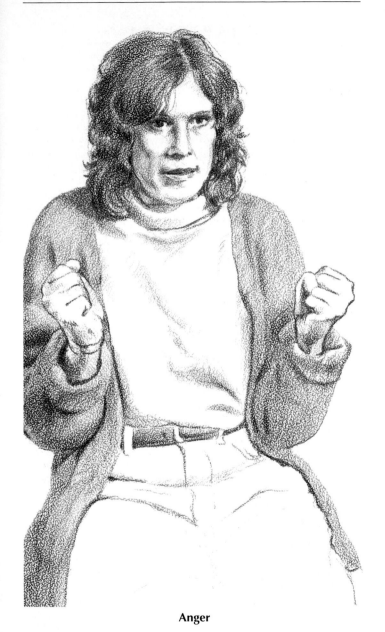

Anger

feelings that we can reflect to our patient. Somehow you have to let the angry person know, without condescension, that you hear him/her and understand how he/she feels, even when the anger is being directed at you. You may have to express your understanding several times before he/she is ready to let go of the anger and move on. Occasionally the person will not want to let go of the anger, even though you have made several attempts to show understanding. In this case you may need to ask what more the patient wants, and how he/she expects you two to work together.

Consider a mild example:

Dr.: Hello, Mr. Limb. How're you doing?

Pt.: Not so hot, Doc. I mean how's a person supposed to park around here? I probably went around the block three times before I found a space. That's why I'm a little late. This is no way to treat sick people, especially people like me with bad hips and knees.

At this point the doctor had better carry out an internal dialogue with himself/herself to avoid an ineffective response.

Dr.: Damn! Another angry person. I hate it when people dump their anger on me.

Internal voice: What are you going to do?

Dr.: Maybe just ignore it.

Internal: That won't work. Remember what Lipp says.

Dr.: Oh yeah. Well, I'll try not to get angry and I will try to tell this jerk that I understand him.

Internal: Jerk?

Dr.: OK, I'll also try to keep my feelings from affecting my behavior with him.

Then,

Dr.: So—you had a really tough time finding anywhere to park.

continued

> **Pt.:** You aren't kidding.
>
> **Dr.:** And it got you upset.
>
> **Pt.:** Pissed me off, to tell the truth.
>
> **Dr.:** Pretty angry. Yeah, I can see how that would be. That would be frustrating. How are you now?
>
> **Pt.:** I'm OK now, Doc. I'll just plan to start a little earlier next time.

3. **An important step in empathizing is determining the source of the anger.** You are probably not that source, but your task includes understanding where the anger comes from.

PROCEDURES

Communicating understanding involves six steps. After you've practiced these in some tough encounters, you may find that fewer are needed; but, it helps to be skilled at using all of them.

1. **Recognize that you are in the presence of a strong feeling.** The most troublesome feelings that we experience in our patients are anger, sadness, fear, and ambivalence. If your patient is angry, you will have to recognize that anger.

2. **Stop the proceedings.** Step back and reflect for a moment on what is happening. You need to identify the strong affect you are experiencing and the underlying feeling the patient has. Is it anger? Sadness? Fear? Something else? If you don't know, you will have to ask. If you think you know, you can advance to the next step.

    You may recognize the anger first by noting your own response. Although we recommend suppressing your own response if it is "anger back," we do believe that an honest response to anger includes some sort of emotional component. We like a version of "Ouch!" Your choice might be "Oh!" or "Wow!" That response may not even be verbalized, but just recognized internally.

3. **Try to name the affect and obtain confirmation from the patient that he/she accepts your understanding.**

> **Dr.:** So Louis, if I'm hearing you right, you're angry about that.

Did you notice the doctor's parenthetic phrase, "if I'm hearing you right"? It is a framing or signposting statement that provides a route into the empathic space. Other framing statements are: "Let me see if I understand you right ...," "If I'm understanding right, you're telling me that ...," "Sounds like ...," the shortest possible framing statement, "So ...," or even an empathic grunt before offering the iterative statement. When the patient adds a correction, you can incorporate it, reiterate your paraphrase and ask for confirmation that you indeed understood correctly.

4. You can then validate the patient's feeling by saying that you can understand it.

> **Dr.:** I see. When you had to go around and around looking for parking past the time for your appointment, you felt pretty angry. I can understand that. If it happened to me, I might be angry, too. And then, on top of all that, my receptionist seemed to be blaming you for the problem, so you were even more upset.

At this point in the empathic process, the patient's affect is no longer so strong because you have been treating the strong affect by understanding it. The underlying problem, both internal and external to the patient, hasn't been remedied; but the immediate affect has been. If this patient is still angry, something remains to be understood. You can ask for more help: "I understand the anger about the parking problem and our receptionist's remark, but you still seem pretty upset and I'm wondering if there is something I don't yet understand." If you've understood the affect, you have received confirmation from your patient (something akin to "You got it, Doc") and you can move on to another subject. You may even get a little praise from your patient for your understanding, something like "At least you understood how it was."

What if the anger doesn't make sense to you? Common reasons that people express anger include fear of the unknown, possibilities of loss (of time, money, comfort, health, control), shame about ignorance, and misdirection—anger at someone or something else gets misdirected at you. Ask questions about how the patient got angry if you don't understand the source of the anger, and listen for these potential causal elements. If you are still baffled, admit it.

> **Dr.:** I'm afraid I am still confused. I heard what you said and can understand that you felt strongly, but I don't yet understand what made you so angry. Can you help me understand this?

continued

> **Pt.:** Doc, this hip and knee pain is really catching up with me. I'm no good for anything anymore.

5. You can also express understanding of actions motivated by strong feelings. If your patient has done something as a result of his/her powerful feeling—like missing an appointment or not taking his/her medicine, or even overdosing as a gesture of sadness—you can offer understanding.

> **Dr.:** I can understand, feeling as you did, how you threw away the pills and didn't go for your x-ray appointment. It makes sense, even if it didn't help your cough much.

6. And you might want to offer help in the future.

> **Dr.** Louis, next time you get upset, maybe we could talk about it and I could try to help more. Could you let me know if you are feeling upset with me? I'd like to be of more help to you.

Offered this approach to the angry patient, physicians express several concerns:

a. Then what? After the empathic response, what do you say or do?
b. Surely there are some people you can't empathize with. You haven't ever been in their shoes. Maybe you don't even like them.
c. Doesn't this take up a terrific amount of time? Where can I find the time to do all this?
d. Isn't this a skill for social workers and psychiatrists? I'm a doctor, not a psychotherapist. Besides, won't empathy just open up the floodgates of patient emotion? Then I'll really be in over my head.

In response to these concerns, we suggest:

a. After the empathic response you do nothing. Don't rush to offer any solution. Just listen and understand. As Weisberg says, "there is no advice for a feeling, no fix for anger, sadness, or fear, just the companionship of understanding" (Weisberg. Does Anybody Listen? Does Anybody Care?, 1995).

To let the understanding do its work, you have to leave a bit of space, perhaps ten seconds. During this pause two things will happen. The patient will feel understood, which is powerfully therapeutic, and your understanding of how this patient is feeling will deepen. Such an understanding will allow you to be more therapeutic to your patient.

b. You can empathize with someone you don't like or with whom you have not shared experiences. Empathy isn't liking or forgiving. Empathy is UNDERSTANDING. You could understand a serial killer if you were able to learn how he/she saw the world even if you didn't like or for-give him/her. Of course you haven't had all your patients' experiences. If you are male, you have never been pregnant. We hope you have never lost a child. But you can still IMAGINE what it might feel like to have your body changing shape, becoming more unwieldy, more foreign to you. You have had losses, and you can imagine that this patient's loss is immensely greater than any you have had.

c. Does empathy take time? Yes, but if you use understanding responses, you will be amazed at how much faster the interview progresses once the emotional outburst is named and understood.

d. Regardless of your specialty, you'll encounter patients' strong feelings. The patient's fears and anger diminish when the physician acknowledges them and tries to understand their source.

7. When the patient is angry about something you did, you must consider whether he/she has a valid case! If so, consider apologizing.

Pt.: Damn it, Doc, you promised you'd be there when I needed the operation. Then when it happened, you were somewhere else. Out playing golf or something.

Dr.: So you felt let down when I wasn't there.

Pt.: You promised, Doc. How am I supposed to trust you?

Dr.: Yeah. You really counted on me and I didn't show up.

Pt.: I was pretty upset. I'm still pretty upset!

continued

Dr.: Well, I can see how you would be. And I think you are right. I owe you an apology. I'm sorry I didn't take more care with my schedule so I could have been there when you needed me. I hope you can forgive me. I'll try hard to do better the next time.

Pt.: Oh, well, ... oh, OK I guess. It's not that I want to hold a grudge.

Dr.: Thanks.

Pt.: Yeah. Thank you too, Doc. I appreciate the apology.

Many complaining patients say that what they want most of all is an apology.

Sometimes we hear stories from our angry patients about another doctor. We may worry that empathizing with our patient's distress will convince the patient that his/her grievance is actionable and that we'll be asked to be a witness in a lawsuit.

Pt.: Five years ago I was in that hospital out in Elsewhere. I was there with a heart attack. My doctor didn't see me for five days. Then he comes and stands in the doorway and says, "Joe, whenever you're sick you go up to the Mayo clinic. Why don't you just go up there now?" I was so mad, I could have torn him apart. If I wasn't hooked up to all those wires and tubes, I would have pounded him into the ground."

Dr.: Was that pain you had five years ago like the pain that got you here today?

This doctor said later that he didn't know how to respond to the patient's anger about his prior doctor. Instead of changing the subject, he might have said:

Dr.: Sounds like you were plenty angry with your doctor back then.

Pt.: Right! Plenty! But I'm over it now. And the doctors here have been really good.

Empathizing is not the same as agreeing with the patient. Empathizing is expressing understanding of how the patient feels.

PITFALLS TO AVOID

1. Failing to recognize the presence of a strong affect: anger, sadness, fear, or the sense of being trapped or caught in a bind.

2. Avoiding empathy because of fear of complications or of "opening Pandora's box."

3. Believing that empathy is some sort of inborn capacity, that you either have or you don't.

PEARL

The best treatment for anger is empathy—understanding.

SELECTED READINGS

Barrett-Lennard GT. The phases and focus of empathy. Br J Med Psychol 1993;66:3–14.

Cohen-Cole SA. The medical interview: the three-function approach. St. Louis: Mosby, 1991.

Egener B. Empathy. In: Feldman MD, Christensen JF, eds. Behavioral medicine for primary care: a practical guide. Stamford, CT: Appleton and Lange, 1997:8–14.

Lipp MR. Respectful Treatment: A practical handbook of patient-care. NY: Elsevier Press, 1986:8.

Olsen DP. Empathy as an ethical and philosophical basis for nursing. ANS Adv Nurs Sci 1991;14:62–75.

Platt FW, Keller VF. Empathic communication: a teachable and learnable skill. J Gen Intern Med 1994;9:222–226.

Platt FW, Platt CM. Empathy, a miracle or nothing at all. JCOM 1998; 5:30–33.

Roter DL, Hall JA, Kern DE, Barker LR, Cole KA, Roca RP. Improving physicians' interviewing skills and reducing patients' emotional distress. A randomized clinical trial. Arch Intern Med 1995;155: 1877–1884.

Smith RC, Hoppe RB. The patient's story: integrating the patient- and physician-centered approaches to interviewing. Ann Intern Med 1991;115:470–477.

Weisberg J. Does anybody listen? does anybody care? Medical Group Management Association, Englewood, CO. 1984:27–38.

CHAPTER 15
Sadness and Fear

PROBLEM

Illness and the process of being cared for provoke strong feelings of shame, humiliation, sadness, and fear in many of our patients. Our patients present these emotions to us. We must be able to work with patients suffering these strong and painful emotions. What do you do when a patient cries? Do you long to escape the interview room? What do you do when a patient expresses his/her worries and terrors? Do you rush to reassure the patient that everything will be fine?

PRINCIPLES

1. **The most effective response to the patient's sadness and fear is empathy.** Listening, confirming what we have heard, and voicing our understanding of the patient's feelings treats the isolation of the patient burdened with strong negative feelings, and it lessens the pain of his/her fear and sadness. We believe, as do Coulehan and Block, that empathy consists of this effort to understand our patients:

   "Empathy is a type of understanding. It is not an emotional state of feeling sympathetic or sorry for someone.
      ...In medical interviewing, being empathic means listening to the total communication—words, feeling, and gestures—and letting the patient know that you are really hearing what he or she is saying. The empathic physician is also the scientific physician because understanding is at the core of objectivity." (Coulehan JL, Block MR. The Medical Interview: Mastering Skills for Clinical Practice. 3rd ed. 1997)

2. **Fear and sadness are not diseases to be cured or injuries to be fixed, but they can be relieved by being understood.**

   "It sounds like you were really frightened when your chest was hurting and you couldn't get relief from the nitro pills."

   "It sounds like you have been full of sadness since your job vanished. You really loved that work."

3. **Strong affects are contagious.** You may find that your responses parallel your patient's and hinder your therapeutic be-

havior. It helps to be aware of your own reciprocal sadness and fear, so your own feelings don't unknowingly influence your interaction with the patient.

PROCEDURES

1. **Realize that you are witnessing the expression of a strong feeling.**

2. **Take time out if you need it to determine which strong feeling you're hearing.** (You can bet that the feeling, if painful, will be some variant of anger, sadness, fear, or ambivalence.)

3. **Try to name the affect for the patient, taking care not to sound confrontational.**
   a) Avoid technical psychosocial terms of diagnosis. If you are dealing with sadness, use that word rather than the clinical "depression." If your patient is fearful you can say, "That sounds like it was scary," or "Sounds like you're pretty fearful about what this all might mean," rather than "You seem to be very anxious." Making a clinical diagnosis out of the feeling is too much, too soon.
   b) Remember the route to the empathic space: start with a framing statement that prepares the patient and you for what is to come. "Mr. F., I need you to stop for a minute. I want to tell you what I've heard so far and then I'd like you to tell me if I got off track. OK?" You are preparing the patient for a brief shift in roles. The patient will now try to understand YOU as you try to understand him/her.
   c) **Empathic communication is part observation, part imagination.** As such, it may miss the point. You have to be prepared for the patient's rejection or correction of your interpretation. If you can't get a pretty clear sense of the patient's feeling, simply ask how he/she feels.

> **Dr.:** I can see that you have some strong feelings about this but I'm not sure exactly what the feeling is. Can you tell me some more about it? For example, what does it make you want to do?

It is the patient you need to understand, but sometimes our own reactions and agendas get in the way of listening, especially when serious or strong concerns are aroused. Being aware of our own thoughts and feelings can help in three ways. First, our feelings can be early clues to what patients themselves are feeling (angry, trapped, bored, or victimized). Using this early warning system for feelings, we can sometimes be more efficient with empathy. Second, acknowledging our ideas and reactions to ourselves keeps them from inadvertently interfering with our judgment and decisions. Finally, explicitly acknowledging our reactions to ourselves instead of denying or suppressing them diminishes our stress, fatigue, and disenchantment with patient care.

Pt.: I was home alone when the pain hit. It got really bad and I took a couple of the nitros but they didn't help. I tried to call my doctor, but his phone line was busy. So I just sat there, and my chest hurt and I couldn't breathe and the sweat was running out of me like my pores had opened up and my soul was seeping out. I thought I was dying. And I took a couple more nitros; you know Dr. Q. had told me not to take more than two or three ever, but it hurt so much. My wife called; she was out shopping and she's worried about me but I didn't want to worry her so I told her I was OK, but I wasn't OK at all. I was really scared.

Dr.: That sounds awful. You were hurting and all alone and ¯ scared.

Pt.: You aren't kidding. I thought I was all done with.

Dr.: So you thought it was the end of you. Yeah, I can imagine.

Pt.: You got it, Doc.

Is that how it really went? No. The doctor, overwhelmed by that powerful story, responded by asking "How long did the chest pain last?" Later, asked why he avoided that strong affective story, he said, "I thought the patient didn't want to talk about it!" Since this patient clearly did talk about his fear, perhaps the doctor was inhibited by his own feelings in listening to this highly charged story.

It's always better to respond to the patient's affect itself. The patient does want to talk about it. The doctor did better with his next patient:

Pt.: It's like I was telling you, Doc. I just have been grieving a lot since I lost my job. I loved that work. I know there were lots of problems with it, but you know, some of the time I felt as if I were fulfilling my destiny. I felt as if I had been cut out to do just that very work. Since I lost it, I've been feeling really sad.

continued

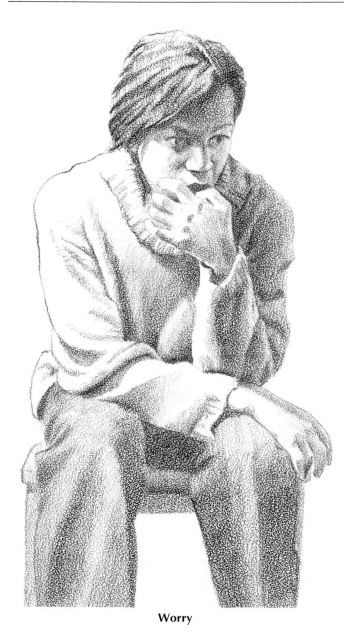

Worry

Dr.: So, if I understand correctly, you have really been sad and grieving since you lost that job.

Pt.: It wasn't perfect.

Dr.: It wasn't perfect, but you still miss it.

Pt.: Yeah.

Dr.: I can understand.

As we try to reflect our understanding of how the patient sees things and how the patient feels, we often miss key components of the story or the patient realizes that he/she still has an important item to add. When the patient adds to or corrects the story, all we have to do is incorporate the correction into our reflective comment. The process itself is immensely therapeutic.

The pause we mentioned in Chapter 14: Anger, is important here as well. When we have understood how our patient is feeling and our patient understands that we understand, the best next step is to stop for a moment, perhaps for five or ten seconds. That magic pause allows two events to take place. First, our patient has a chance to relish being understood and to feel better. Second, we have a chance to digest what it might feel like to feel as our patient does right now.

4. **Validate the feeling.** "I can understand. It makes sense to me that you feel that way."

5. **Accept or understand your patient's actions that were based on that feeling.**

6. **Offer help in the future.** We can also empathize with our patient's successes, joys, enthusiasms, and achievements. "Sounds like your making that trip despite your MS was important to you and you showed you could do it. That must feel good!"

PITFALLS TO AVOID

1. Becoming overwhelmed by the patient's strong sadness or fear and avoiding any response to his/her feelings.

2. Trying to reassure or comfort the patient before showing understanding.

3. Not trying to understand the patient because you don't like him/her or have never had such an experience.

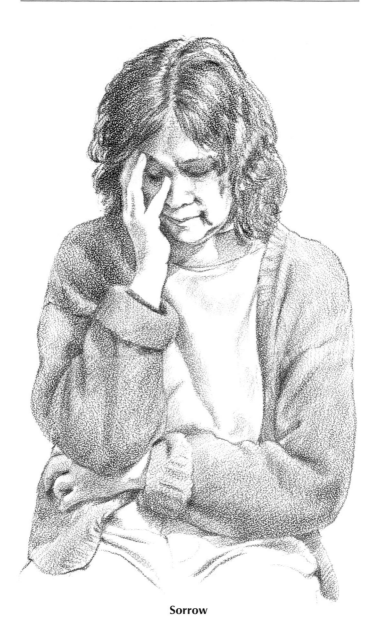

Sorrow

4. Going through the reflective process mechanically without pause or imagination.

PEARL

Empathy assuages the strong feelings you cannot fix.

SELECTED READINGS

Berger J, Mohr J. A fortunate man. London: Penguin Press, 1967.

Brunton SA, Radecki SE. Teaching physicians to be patient: a hospital admission experience for family practice residents. J Am Board Fam Pract 1992;5:581–588.

Cohen-Cole SA. The medical interview: the three-function approach. St. Louis: Mosby Year Book, 1991.

Coulehan JL, Block MR. The medical interview: mastering skills for clinical practice. 3rd ed. Philadelphia: FA Davis, 1997.

Covey SR. Habit 5: seek first to understand, then to be understood. In: The seven habits of highly effective people. NY: Simon and Schuster, 1986.

Haerlin A. The doctor–patient relationship. Medical Encounter. Spring 1998;14:19–21.

Lazare A. Shame and humiliation in the medical encounter. Arch Intern Med 1987;147:1653–1568.

Novack DH, Suchman AL, Clark W et al. Calibrating the physician: personal awareness and effective patient care. JAMA 1997;278:502–509.

Suchman AL, Markakis K, Beckman HB, Frankel R. A Model of empathic communication in the medical interview. JAMA. 1997;277:678–682.

Sullivan HS. The collected works of Harry Stack Sullivan. NY: Norton, 1964.

CHAPTER 16
Ambivalence

PROBLEM

What we call "denial" and "resistance" may largely be artifacts of our approach to interviewing. If so, we can abandon our old approach and try a new one.

> **Dr.:** You have to quit smoking. It's killing you.
>
> **Pt.:** It's not a problem.
>
> **Dr. (aside):** He/she is *in denial* and *resists* all my efforts to help.

New information about how people change offers us a way of understanding patients' persistence in life-threatening behaviors despite our attempts to bully and cajole them into health. Studies done at drug and alcohol treatment centers describe behavior change as a continuum through which people move with or without our help.

Prochaska and his colleagues found that most people go through a similar series of stages as they change any behaviors: precontemplative, contemplative, planning, action, maintenance, and identification (Prochaska JO, Norcross JC, Diclemente CC. Changing for Good: a Revolutionary Six-Stage Program for Overcoming Bad Habits and Moving Your Life Positively Forward, 1994). People can relapse at any stage or make a slip (a deviation smaller than a relapse).

All of us start out in a *precontemplative* stage, unaware of the behavior or that any change is needed. When we label patients "irresponsible," we are usually talking about people in the precontemplative stage. Their risky health behavior isn't a problem for which they take responsibility, because they don't yet see it as a problem. A precontemplative smoker, for example, might say that "smoking is not a problem for me and isn't going to be one. That health stuff is malarkey. It's a problem for my wife—she's after me to quit—not for me." Of course, it's hard to find a precontemplative smoker in the U.S. these days.

Most of us move on to a *contemplative* or *ambivalent* stage. Dabbling at change identifies this ambivalent or contemplative stage wherein we weigh the alternatives and keep trying to decide which way to go. A person can be ambivalent for a long time. The ambivalent person demonstrates his/her bind with a two-handed gesture, "on the one hand, and on the other hand." A contemplative smoker might tell you all the reasons to quit (to avoid cancer, to please my spouse and kids, to get rid of this chronic cough, because it has become an unsocial

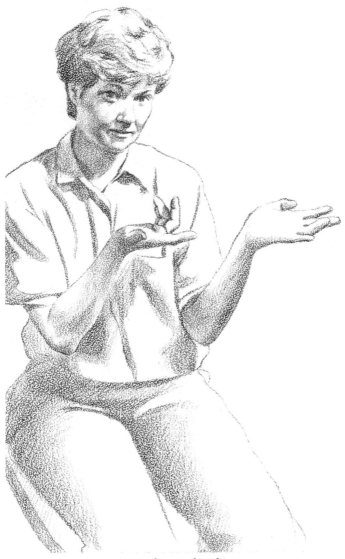

"On the one hand"

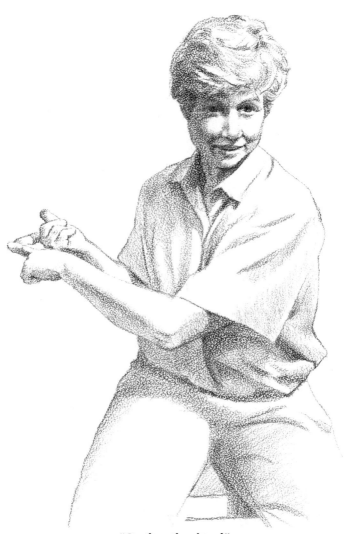

"On the other hand"

thing to do ...) and then add all the reasons to continue smoking (smoking helps me deal with stress at work, helps me focus my thoughts, keeps me slender ...).

If we're able to move out of the contemplative stage, we may progress to *planning*, *action*, *maintenance,* and eventually *identification* with the new life style.

If you ask your patient to tell you his/her thoughts about a behavior you consider a threat to the patient's health, most likely he/she will tell you of his/her ambivalence. That's where most of our patients are. You can respond with understanding of that "stuck" state.

> **Dr.:** I see. Sounds like you're feeling ambivalent about this. A lot of reasons to quit and a lot of reasons to continue. You're kind of stuck there.
>
> **Pt.:** I am, Doc. I've been planning to do something about it for a long time.
>
> **Dr:** I can understand.

Once you recognize the "stuck" state, you're ready to begin working as an agent of change. You can start by asking if the patient sees any way that you can help him/her get unstuck.

PRINCIPLES

1. Many of our patients who seem irresponsible, in denial, or resistant to our advice about their unhealthy habits are stuck in an ambivalent state. **The best tool for working with ambivalence is empathy, an understanding response.**

2. We can increase the patient's denial and resistance through our interviewing techniques. Pleading, threatening, or leaning on someone almost always engenders resistance, a reaction in the opposite direction. What looks like denial to us may simply be the result of the patient's cost : benefit analysis differing from ours.

3. The ambivalent state is enormously powerful, perhaps because the known evil is easier to tolerate than the unknown evil. **People can remain ambivalent for a very long time.**

4. Once your patient feels understood and not oppressed by you, he/she will feel freer to accept your help in making a change.

5. Moving beyond a contemplative stage requires planning for the next step. **It is especially important to help the patient plan replacements for the pleasures they will lose with the change in behavior.**

6. Only about 20% of your patients who are considering a major be-
    havior change are in the action phase and thus responsive to your
    suggestions about what to do and how to do it. **Don't waste your
    time giving advice to someone who isn't ready for it.**

7. In order for people to move from one stage to another, they need
    conviction that the change is important and confidence that they
    can do it. They first have to see the cost:benefit ratio favoring
    change and see that they possess the tools to do it.

PROCEDURES

1. Determine the patient's state of change by describing the stages
    and asking your patient to tell you where he/she is on the contin-
    uum. **Reiterate the patient's explanation, checking for accu-
    racy.**

> **Dr.:** So it sounds like you are in a bind, caught between two
> attractive alternatives. Sounds like you're feeling ambivalent
> about smoking.

2. Maintain a posture of balanced curiosity—eagerness and willing-
    ness to hear what the patient has to say. **Avoid argumentation.**

3. To learn as much as you can about how the patient views the be-
    havior, **ask the patient to tell you the good points of the harm-
    ful behavior.**

> **Dr.:** Roger, tell me the good things about smoking.
>
> **Pt.:** What do you mean, "good things"? There aren't any. It's
> just a dirty habit.
>
> **Dr.:** Hmm. I doubt that. You wouldn't be doing it if there was-
> n't anything good about it. For example, do you like the taste?
>
> **Pt.:** Yeah. It does give me pleasure.
>
> **Dr.:** I see. What else?
>
> **Pt.:** Well, it helps with the stress at work. Sometimes I have to
> take a break and light up and then I feel calmer.
>
> **Dr.:** What else?
>
> *continued*

Pt.: Keeps me from bloating out. If I quit, I eat like a pig.

Dr.: So pleasure, help with work stress, preventing obesity—what else?

Pt.: That's it, Doc.

Why get the patient to list the good features? Why stress the cons of change? Aren't you supposed to be convincing the patient to change? No, you aren't. **You're supposed to be finding out where the patient stands on the issue of change.** Then he/she will convince you.

Dr.: So it sounds like there are several good reasons to continue smoking.

Pt.: Well, yeah, but I'm no dope, you know. I watch TV. I know there's a lot of good reasons to quit too.

Dr.: Oh? Like what?

Pt.: Well my health for one. And my kids are on my case to quit. So's my wife. And the boss doesn't really like our taking time off to smoke. And I got this cough all the time and I know my lungs aren't doing so hot. I puff when I walk up stairs.

If you listen to the patient's whole story, your patient will choose where he/she wants the balance to fall. Now you won't be hearing "Yes, but" from the patient. He/she will have generated the list of pros and cons that you can discuss and won't feel as if you were against him/her but able to work together on this issue. To confirm that you are indeed right there with the patient, you can empathize with the dilemma.

Dr.: So, if I understand you right, you are really caught in a dilemma. You have a bunch of reasons to quit smoking and another bunch to keep on. That's a tough spot to be in.

Pt.: You aren't kidding, Doc. I feel trapped.

Dr.: Trapped. Yeah, I see how that would be.

4. **Plot the patient's decision point.** This useful staging technique, devised by Keller and Kemp-White, consists of rating the answers to two questions on a scale of one to ten. **"How convinced**

are you that this behavior change is important to you?" and "How confident are you that you can make this change?" The result is a Cartesian plot of the patient's decision point. Knowing where your patient is, in relation to these two questions, will allow you to tailor your therapeutic response. A patient who is unconvinced may need to see data. A convinced but unconfident patient may need help planning simple steps toward change.

> **Dr.:** John, your diabetes seems out of control. Your blood sugar today was 350, your A1C last week was 14%, and you tell me you aren't even testing your blood sugars. What's going on?
>
> **Dr.:** You're right, Doctor. I just hate sticking my finger. I can't even stand the sight of blood. And my old glucometer is a mess. I don't think it works anymore.

The doctor and the patient had been working together for fifteen years. The patient, an intelligent, articulate, scientifically trained 45-year-old professional, had made his own diagnosis of diabetes 10 years ago and treatment with insulin twice a day had initially seemed successful. Lately things were going awry. The doctor thought his patient's explanation could lead to remedy: a spring-loaded finger-sticking device and a new, simpler glucometer. But this doctor had recently learned of the two key questions about conviction and confidence.

> **Dr.:** John, just for the fun of it, I'd like to ask you two questions. On a scale of one to ten, how convinced are you of the importance of tight control of your blood sugars?
>
> **Pt.:** About two. I figure something will eventually kill me, maybe the diabetes. I doubt that I have much to do with it.
>
> **Dr.:** Wow! That's a surprise. Well, just for the fun of it, if you were convinced, how confident would you be that you could do what it takes to control the sugars?
>
> **Pt.:** Oh, it would be a snap. Those were just excuses.

The doctor said that he was surprised. He expected this patient to be convinced but not confident. He found the opposite. Instead of small steps, he offered some medical literature. The patient read, became convinced, and blood sugars improved.

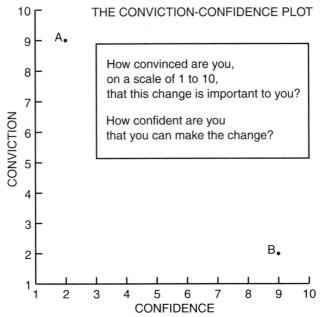

A: Initial Expectation of Physician. B: Patient's actual position.

5. **If you continue to care for patients who do not accept your recommendations for behavior change, document your ideas, intent, and conversations in the medical chart.** Staging and conviction–confidence plots can be part of this documentation.

6. **Move your patient along one stage at a time.** Try to get your precontemplative patient thinking about the issue. Try to get your ambivalent contemplator making some plans.

7. To increase conviction: ask permission to bring new health information to your patient's attention; personalize information to the patient's status; clarify the hierarchy of your patient's values and reflect them back to him/her; be curious and ask about patient behavior that seems inconsistent with his/her values.

8. To increase confidence: recall other challenges the patient has overcome; break large tasks into small, do-able chunks; make the first steps easy to ensure early success; have patients reward themselves for successes; and involve social supports, families, and friends.

PITFALLS TO AVOID

1. Telling your patient what to do despite evidence that it doesn't work.

2. Expecting miracles. Believing that all patients, not just those with acute myocardial infarction or the diagnosis of a cancer, will jump from precontemplation to action.

3. Arguing, exhorting, and trying to scare your patient, engendering resistance and denial.

4. Failing to understand where your patient is on the change spectrum or the conviction–confidence plot.

PEARL

You can help your patient if you work hard to understand how things look to him/her and then use proven strategies to help the patient move to the next stage of change.

SELECTED READINGS

Bandura A. Self-efficiency: toward a unifying theory of behavioral change. Psychol Rev 1977;84:191–215.

Keller VF, Kemp-White M. Choices and changes: a new model for influencing patient health behavior. JCOM 1997;4(6):33–36.

Marlatt GA, Gordon JR. editors. Relapse prevention: maintenance strategies in the treatment of addictive behaviors. NY: Guilford Press, 1985.

Miller WR, Rollnick S. Motivational interviewing: preparing people to change addictive behavior. NY: Guillford Press, 1991.

Prochaska JO, Norcross JC, Diclemente CC. Changing for good: a revolutionary six-stage program for overcoming bad habits and moving your life positively forward. NY: Avon Books, 1994.

CHAPTER 17

Giving Bad News

PROBLEM

Most of us find it difficult to give bad news to our patients. Some doctors avoid giving bad news by asking someone else to do it. Others deliver the news, then flee before the patient has a chance to assimilate it and start expressing feelings or asking questions. Still others understand that communicating bad news demands the same skills that we need in discussing other health matters.

PRINCIPLES

1. A lot of our contact with patients occurs when things are not going well in their lives. If you are going to be a complete physician, you have to be able to give bad news in a therapeutic way.

2. When we fail at giving bad news therapeutically, it may be because our own feelings get in the way. The situation may stir up our own sadness, anger, or anxiety, blocking our ability to function as therapeutic physicians.

3. The patient's response to a diagnosis may not make sense to us. One patient may respond to our report that we are unable to treat his/her viral upper respiratory disease with the same degree of passion another displays when given a diagnosis of carcinomatosis. Whether the effect of our bad news is long- or short-term, our patients experience disappointment as a result of what we have told them, and we must be prepared to receive those feelings in a way that will be helpful to the patient.

PROCEDURES

1. **Be prepared.** Although the interaction cannot be controlled, you can rehearse the beginning of the interview and identify some of the outcomes you desire. It helps to go over some of the words you plan to use and to anticipate your listener's likely questions and reactions.

2. **Start with yourself.** Preparing yourself mentally to give bad news is an important step in the encounter. Doctors may be particularly sensitive to the failure of medicine or of the body to cure itself, and our sense of failure is magnified when we have to explain it to people who have come to us for help. If we are fond

of them, we feel even worse. On top of feelings of inadequacy, we are being threatened with loss. Wanting to avoid feeling these feelings is normal; but when we try, we abdicate our power and do damage to the patient in the process.

We get other feelings from having to give bad news. For example, we dread telling a patient that he/she has a viral URI when the patient has been insisting on an antibiotic. The doctor may be wishing he/she didn't have to spend more time explaining a URI than explaining a cancer. However, the doctor must get past his/her annoyance before talking to the patient.

Sometimes the bad news we have to impart is that we have erred. We have to find a way to say, "I made a mistake." Suppose, for example, that your office has overlooked an abnormal Pap smear, only noting it 8 months later. The patient's dysplasia has probably advanced, causing a need for more extensive surgery, and perhaps making curative treatment impossible. Most of us would be feeling guilty, incompetent, and frightened. We would be wishing for some way to protect ourselves from what we imagine will be the patient's anger and desire for retribution. Such a combination of guilt, embarrassment, and fear makes it hard for the doctor to talk with the patient; yet in order to have a therapeutic encounter, the physician must acknowledge those feelings and put them aside to concentrate on the patient's needs.

The task of sorting out your own emotional responses, acknowledging them to yourself, and getting them under control may take a minute or two. Experience and practice help you to get through the process more easily, and studies show that patients appreciate the bearer of bad news sharing some feelings about it. When we are aware of our feelings and honor them, we can get past our natural desire for self-protection and move into the therapeutic role.

3. **Think about the setting.** You will need some privacy. If a family member will be present with your patient, you may benefit from having a colleague present, too. If you bring an ally, coach that person ahead of time on what you want from him/her. You can use the silent observer to check out your perceptions about what was said and understood during the encounter. You might also use the observer as a monitor of your own performance, first explaining your feelings and how you plan to manage the interaction.

Think of this encounter as a medical procedure, and allow a block of time just as you might for a flexible sigmoidoscopy. You will need time to sit silently with your patient so he/she can assimilate the news and ask questions. As the listeners take in more of the bad news, you will probably have to repeat your explanations. Be prepared for phone calls after the interview.

Giving bad news is a process, not a single event. You can schedule another visit in a week or so to continue. As the patient begins to think about the bad news and tell others, he/she will have more questions.

4. **Prepare the patient—give warning.** In setting the appointment, give the patient some preparation for bad news to come. If you are unsure of the diagnosis but think that it might be something life-threatening like cancer, mention that diagnosis along with other possible diagnoses, explaining that you need to investigate further to be sure which is the true problem. This survey of possibilities lays the groundwork for a subsequent conversation, if indeed the worst proves to be true.

When asking the patient to come in, you need an introductory sentence, perhaps something like, "I've found a problem, and I want to spend some time talking with you about it." You can say that some people like detailed information and some just want the big picture, then ask "What would you like?" You may suggest that some people find it helpful to have company when they're talking about health matters that might be complicated, and ask if the patient would like his/her spouse (daughter, son, father, mother...) to be present.

5. **Start by finding out what the patient knows, what the patient thinks is happening, and what concerns or fears he/she has.** With bad news, the physician is tempted to start talking right away. It's better to start listening.

Dr.: Before we start [actually this **IS** starting] I want to ask you what you know about this problem you have and what you have been thinking about it.

Pt.: I don't know, Doctor. That's why I came to you.

Most patients will eagerly provide you with their own ideas, concerns, or expectations. Some need a bit more prompting.

Dr.: Well, OK. But I know you probably had some thoughts about what might be going on.

Pt.: I guess I was worried that I had some sort of infection.

In order to deliver your news effectively, you need to understand your patient's assumptions about his/her illness.

Almost every sufferer who comes to a healer in any society comes with an explanatory model, i.e., a combination of ideas about diagnosis, causation, and potential therapy. We can discover those ideas by asking, and if we fail to ask, we handicap ourselves in our further discussion with the patient. At the very least, our patient will be asking himself/herself why we haven't considered what the patient thinks is the most likely explanation.

You can also ask what questions the patient most wants answered.

Then you are ready to start your explanation. You will need to use short sentences and tailor your vocabulary to your patient. Leave pauses so the patient can absorb what you are telling him.

Dr.: Well, John, the news is really worse than that. We now know that it isn't an infection, it's a cancer.

(pause)

Dr.: We've found that that lung patch we were worried about is really a cancer instead of a pneumonia.

(pause)

Pt.: You said it's a cancer?

Dr.: Yes, it is.

Pt.: That means the end of me, doesn't it?

Dr.: Is that how the news sounds? Like it's all over?

Pt.: Well, cancer—you know.

Dr.: Not necessarily. Tell me what that word means to you. Different people understand it differently.

Even in the middle of giving the bad news, you are finding out about your patient while giving him/her information. Your patient's response to bad news may be anger, fear, denial, or a combination of these. **Your job is to hear the patient's response, to stay with him/her, and to express your understanding of how the diagnosis sounds and feels to the patient, while being prepared to repeat yourself until the patient has finished his/her questions during this encounter.**

6. **Plan to repeat yourself.** Remember that the patient or his/her companion rarely hears the details of the bad news the first time you give them. You can safely assume that once the essential fact—"It's cancer," "It's Alzheimer's," is given, the patient will

probably hear nothing further. Bad news usually induces temporary mental paralysis.

You can expect little of what you first said to be retained. So it helps to ask for feedback after you think you have told what you came to tell, divulged the bad news, and explained everything. You can say that sometimes, talking about complex issues like this, you have found that your explanations are not clear. To be sure you said it clearly, you'd like your patient to tell you what he/she heard.

If you schedule another visit to rediscuss the matter, at that time it might be helpful to give the patient additional resources. These could be written materials, pamphlets provided by various organizations, audiotapes of the prior visit, and referrals to patient groups or sometimes to another patient of yours who has this disease and is willing to share the experience of living with it.

Giving bad news is an iterative process. You find out where your patient is, tell a little, wait a while, listen to the reaction, wait again, then start over again. How many times? As many it takes.

You may want to inquire about other people your patient would like to have informed, other people who are available to support your patient, and who else your patient wants involved at the next explanation.

7. **Include hopeful information with the bad news.** Despite the pain and fear that bad news induces, the doctor can help the patient by learning what gives the patient hope and supporting those resources. You can ask, "What's really important to you now and how can we maximize your ability to do what you want to do?" Having a fatal illness is one thing. Thinking that you won't be able to make it to your favorite grandson's graduation is another. We may be able to provide hope in the important small things of life. Some patients find consolation in religion, and most patients find hope in the doctor's promise to stick with them throughout their travails.

Some people who receive bad news become deeply depressed and even suicidal. You can let your patient know that such a response is possible and that you will be available to help in such a circumstance. "We can talk about it" is an offer that engenders hope.

Sometimes humor and hope live together. Humor may raise its cheerful head in the worst circumstances. Your patient may use humor as an ego defense. You can appreciate his/her efforts, but it is usually not appropriate for you to be the jesting one. People expect the doctor to take the illness seriously, whether the patient appears to or not.

8. **Take your time.** The most important skill in offering hope, an important part of giving bad news, is to take your time. Let the

bad news percolate through first. Let the patient tell you his/her worst fears, and deepest sense of loss and grief. Don't try to reassure with hope before you and the patient have fully assimilated the bad news. Hope offered too quickly will be perceived as false hope, minimizing the patient's feelings.

> **Dr.:** So, in short, you have cancer.
>
> **Pt.:** Oh my God! Oh my God!
>
> **Dr.:** But we have some terrifically effective chemotherapy for this sort of tumor.
>
> **Pt.:** Oh my God, Oh me, oh me!

The diagnosis was given and the dialogue proved ineffective. Reassurance in the face of bad news discounts the patient's valid shock and fear. Sometimes reassurance carries a worse message: "Things aren't as bad as you SAY they are." This is even more discounting. To avoid sounding glib, postpone your reassurances until the patient can hear them, and then only promise what you are sure you can deliver. **If the reassurance is to instill hope, it must wait its turn and be modest.**

9. **Know good news when you see it.** Giving good news can't be a problem, can it? But consider those conversations when the doctor, diligently searching for terrible pathology, finds none and cannot seem to switch gears from "failure to find out what's wrong" to "I have good news for you; we haven't found any serious problem." The author recalls overhearing a neurosurgical resident in the emergency room telling two parents that he hadn't found any abnormality on their little son's head CT scan. His "We couldn't find anything. The scan was negative," was delivered with such despair that the parents, sensing his distress, became more distressed themselves. We have to be able to recognize good news, even if it doesn't solve our diagnostic problems.

The ER doctor could tell the parents that he has good news, then point out that this still doesn't explain the child's difficulty, but they can have some assurance that it isn't a brain tumor.

If worried about that possibility, wouldn't you feel better hearing the problem wasn't a brain tumor?

Delivering good news in a grudging manner probably occurs most frequently when we give patients information, especially results of tests, that is "negative." In our zealous search for the disease causing the trouble, the absence of a clear diagnosis is bad news to us. We have to remember that it can be good news to our patients.

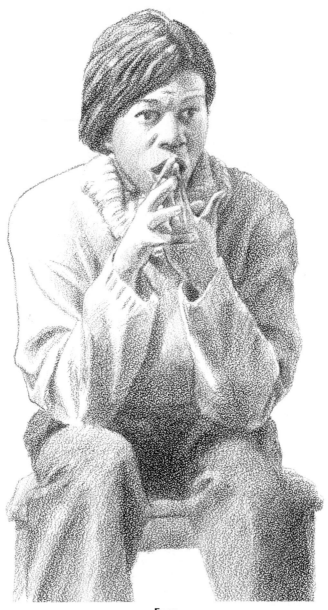

Fear

PITFALLS TO AVOID

1. Failing to prepare.

2. Failing to identify and understand your own feelings and how they might affect your interaction with the patient.

3. Rushing through the encounter, covering your agenda, then leaving the patient and his/her companion to call if they have any further questions.

4. Failing to ask the patient to describe his/her concerns and ideas about the illness.

5. Failing to realize how little information the patient retains from the first shocking conversation with you.

PEARL

The process of giving bad news starts with acknowledging your own reactions to the news, then putting them aside in order to help the patient.

SELECTED READINGS

Brewin TB. Three ways of giving bad news. *Lancet* 1991;337: 1207–1212.

Buckman R. How to break bad news: a guide for health care professionals. J. Hopkins Press: Baltimore, 1992.

Fallowfield LJ, Lipkin M. Delivering sad or bad news. In: Lipkin M, Putnam SM, Lazare A, eds. The medical interview. clinical care, education and research. NY: Springer-Verlag, 1995:316–323.

Novack DH, Suchman AL, Clark W, Epstein RM, Majberg E, Kaplan C. Calibrating the physician: personal awareness and effective patient care. JAMA 1997;278:502–509.

Placek JT, Eberhardt TL. Breaking bad news: a review of the literature. *JAMA* 1996:276:496–502.

Quill TE, Townsend P. Bad news: delivery, dialogue, dilemmas. Arch Intern Med 1991;151:463–468.

Reiser SJ. Words as scalpels: transmitting evidence in the clinical dialogue. Ann Intern Med 1980:92:837–842.

CHAPTER 18
Comforting the Grieving Family

PROBLEM

Some of our most difficult conversations are those with a fearful or grieving family. We may believe that we have little or no hope to offer. Yet to be therapeutic we must focus on the survivors, who need our attention in their suffering. The grieving family is a separate entity from their deceased relative.

PRINCIPLES

1. This encounter may have features in common with the new patient interview: you may have had no previous connection with the family and may never have known the patient before the disaster.

2. Attention to the survivors' grief after notification of a death comes before any explanations of your biomedical search for diagnoses and therapy.

3. Although you will want to observe some basic practices, no approach fits all surviving families. Some may have cultural rituals and beliefs about death and the dead body that are foreign to you. You may need to call on the expertise of a person familiar with the culture of the deceased to be sure you can meet the family's needs.

4. Some responses and concerns are common to most families that have lost a member:
   Cognitive responses include
   a) "Could I or anyone have done anything to prevent this?" and
   b) "Was he/she alone? Was he/she in pain? Did he/she suffer?"

   Emotional responses range from shut-down, "shock," and numbness, to despair, wailing, and anger. Sometimes the survivors will displace their feelings to you, the messenger.

5. If you are to continue caring for members of the bereaved family, a gesture of sympathy—going to the funeral or even a sympathy card—may be helpful. The physician can be aware that grieving is a process, and check to see how his/her patients are handling the loss in subsequent visits.

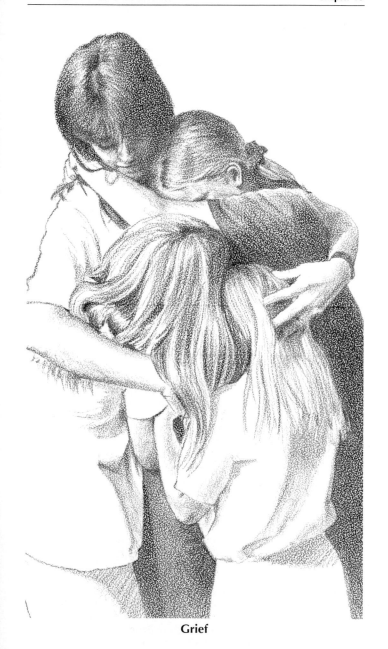

Grief

PROCEDURES

1. As you do when delivering all bad news, **plan ahead.** You must sort out your own feelings, considering what you plan to say and how you plan to say it. Find a protected environment, prepare the listeners, and plan to spend some time.

2. **Find out who is who.** Understand who you are talking with. Do what is necessary to control the setting. Introduce yourself and any colleagues who are present.

3. **Say that you have bad news.** Tell the bad news. Leave pauses to allow people to react and respond, both cognitively and emotionally. If one of the responses is missing, you may give permission for its expression. Grief includes some demonstrations of emotion. There may be tears, wails, and more physical activity than you are comfortable with. Your task is to sit still, to remain present, to avoid trying to fix anything. Your task is to stay with the grieving person, physically and cognitively, perhaps even emotionally. **Don't run away.**

4. If the family wants to spend time with the person who died, perhaps alone, see that their wishes are accommodated.

5. Ask about the family's needs in an empathic way.

> **Dr.:** I've never had such a terrible thing happen in my life, but I can imagine that this is probably one of the worst things you've had to go through.
>
> **Mother:** You can't imagine, Doctor. You just can't imagine.
>
> **Dr.:** No. Probably you've never imagined anything so terrible happening to you, either.
>
> **Mother:** I just can't believe it. He was so alive, just this morning. He asked me to bake him a pie. I can't believe he's dead.
>
> **Dr.:** I know. Unbelievable. Do you have someone who can stay with you tonight, Mrs. A.? It might be hard to drive home from the hospital by yourself. Can I call someone for you?

6. If you were not involved with the patient before his/her death, find out who the patient was. What sort of a person was the patient? What were his/her interests and personal characteristics?
   You can say, "I never knew Barbara before this disaster. Can you tell me a little about who she was, what sort of a person? The grieving family will usually want to do this, to remember the

person they have lost, to recount his/her personal characteristics, voice, thoughts, phrases, behaviors. It will be therapeutic to the family for you to ask about the patient.

7. Resist any anxious desire to cut off the display of emotion by explanations or technical talk.

8. Tread gently on matters relating to the disposition of the body. The survivors may have cultural and religious rituals they want to observe.

9. You may plan to ask about organ donation. Be gentle.

> **Dr.:** I know this is a terrible time for you. Some people find comfort in giving a gift of an organ to help another. Sort of a way to have some good to come out of the tragedy. Did Jimmy ever talk about this?

10. Warn the bereaved of features of grief. Sleeplessness, wild imagining, or hearing or seeing the lost person are all possible. Some, on getting terrible news, are at risk of suicide. **Offer help.**

PITFALLS TO AVOID

1. Running away from the grieving people, thinking you can do nothing.

2. Trying to use the same discourse you would use when discussing a patient with a colleague, discussing loss in biomedical terms as opposed to the emotional language of loss.

> **Dr.:** The problem was that she was exsanguinated. By the time we got her, her myocardium and her brain had been anoxic for too long and the resuscitation couldn't succeed. We tried volume and pressors, even a G-suit.
>
> **Grieving mother:** I can't believe she's dead. Oh no, she left home only about an hour ago.

3. Going into the meeting with your own feelings still unassayed and becoming overwhelmed by them when you least expect it.

4. Viewing the death as a minor mishap en route to organ donation or an autopsy, and rushing to ask for those permissions before the family has digested the bad news and had some time to grieve.

5. Expressing astonishment or revulsion at the surviving family's expectations about death and how one cares for the body.

PEARL

Attend to the grieving survivors. They are now your patients, and they are suffering from a terrible loss.

SELECTED READINGS

Klessig J. Dying the good death. Death and culture: the multicultural challenge. Ann Long-term Care 1998;6:285–290.

Lazare A. Bereavement. In: Lipkin M, Putnam SM, Lazare A, eds. The medical interview. clinical care, education and research. NY: Springer-Verlag, 1995:324–330.

Lindeman E. Symptomatology and management of acute grief. Am J Psychiatry. 1944;101:141–148.

Middleton W, Raphael B. Bereavement; the state of the art and the state of the science. Psychiatric Clin N Am 1987;10:329–343.

Quill TE. A midwife through the dying process: stories of healing and hard choices at the end of life. Baltimore: Johns Hopkins Univ. Press, 1996.

Tolle SW, Elliot DL, Girard DE. How to manage patient death and care for the bereaved. Postgrad Med 1985;78:87–89, 92–95.

Part IV

Illness and Loss

CHAPTER 19
Somatization

PROBLEM

Patients who present with symptoms that you cannot place in a diagnosis, symptoms that find little support in the physical examination and laboratory tests, symptoms that just won't go away and may be highly personalized and idiosyncratic, are especially troublesome.

Kroenke noted that, of the ten most common symptoms in primary care, we find a diagnosis in only about 30%. Most of the patients whose symptoms we can't diagnose are comforted by our failure to find anything seriously wrong, but about 10% are still distressed. Somatization patients display the classic triad of a) undiagnosed physical symptoms, b) psychosocial stress or a psychiatric disorder that the patient doesn't recognize, and c) high health-care utilization. The concept of somatization, and the linked concept of somatoform disorder, now includes many of the patients previously classified as suffering from hypochondriacism, psychosomatic illnesses, and hysteria. The somatizing patient raises several difficult questions for doctors:

- Does the patient have a disease we have failed to diagnose? Are the symptoms out of proportion to the evidence of disease? (In most diseases there is poor correlation between symptoms and the objective findings, so this distinction may be of little help.)
- Is this one of those illnesses that will vanish before we ever reach a diagnosis, at which point we can breathe a sigh of relief, or is it an early presentation of a disease that progresses and will be recognizable later?
- Is this a disorder that will never yield to a clear biomedical or psychosocial diagnosis, but will remain forever to plague the patient and puzzle the doctor?
- How can we make our understanding of the psychological component of symptoms meaningful and acceptable to the patient?

For both patient and physician, the central issue is **uncertainty.** Both want to name the illness and to find remedies. The patient may have collected a number of diagnoses in his/her trip from doctor to doctor, but found no remedy. You cannot leap to any conclusions about this patient's symptoms because of your adherence to methods of observation and testing. Thus you both must remain in a state of uncertainty, an uncomfortable position for both of you.

PRINCIPLES

1. Patients with symptoms in excess of findings, no clear diagnosis, comorbid psychosocial distress or disorders that they minimize,

115

and high use of medical services are the 10% of your patients that take up 50% of your time. They are the ultimate test of our mettle.

2. We cannot deal well with somatizing patients without being conscious of our feelings toward them and making an effort to keep those feelings from affecting our care of the patient. If we act out of those feelings, we may make a tough situation even worse.

3. Chronic or recurrent somatization does not fit well with our acute illness model. A better way to view it is as a chronic disability. Most of these patients may be presenting a psychological problem in a somatized form, but the underlying emotional issues or disorders may not be evident to the patient.

4. In treating somatization, it helps to think of the patient's problem as a puzzle in mind–body linkage. Physical and psychological symptoms are pieces of a puzzle that, together with other pieces, may provide a clearer picture of the patient's illness. Patients with somatization should be evaluated for physical illness, but are also at great risk for escalating procedures and iatrogenic illness.

PROCEDURES

1. Assume that uncertainty is an inevitable part of the medium in which physicians do their work. We will not be able to diagnose many of the problems patients bring us, and may be surprised in a number of cases where we thought we had everything figured out.

2. **Try to legitimize your patient's experience** and empathize with it.

> **Dr.:** Mr S., even though we haven't found a specific cause of your pain, I can see that it's a major problem for you. I believe that you have been suffering a great deal. You know, feeling as bad as you do and still not knowing what to do about it must be really frustrating. I can understand how tough it must be.

3. **Try to elicit your patient's ideas about causes and expectations for further investigation and treatment.**

> **Dr.:** Tell me what you think is wrong and what needs to be done about it.

continued

> **Pt.:** I don't know. That's why I've come to you.
>
> **Dr.:** Yes. But I'd like to know what you're most concerned about. What have you already learned about this symptom? Does anyone else you know have something like this? What were you hoping I could do to help?

4. Adopt a slower pace with this patient, reformulate treatment goals, schedule regular visits, and be alert to ways in which the symptoms might link with psychological conditions. The pace or tempo of care of somatizing patients is slower than that of patients with most other conditions, and requires a continuous relationship, often over years. Thus it is hard for most residents to experience in most training programs. Few psychiatrists have much experience with unexplained physical symptoms either, so our usual consultants may be unversed in this area of concern.

   While remaining vigilant for objective evidence of diseases that explain the symptoms, **try shifting treatment goals to rehabilitation, or maintaining or regaining function.**

> **Dr.:** Mr. S., until we can find a specific treatment for your symptoms, we need to help you (keep your job, stay in school, take care of yourself at home ....)

   If this is a patient who also discovers his/her direst needs at night or on weekends, the doctor can incorporate regular visits as part of the rehabilitation plan, discouraging urgent calls.
   You must also look for psychiatric syndromes often associated with somatization: alcohol and drug use, depression, anxiety, and a history of physical or sexual abuse.

5. **Focus on function.** Ask, "How has this set of symptoms affected the rest of your life?" and address the problems contained in the answer. The **BATHE mnemonic** suggests that you inquire about **Background** ("What is going on in your life?"), **Affect** ("How do you feel about it?"), **Trouble** ("What troubles you the most about this situation?"), **Handle** ("What helps you handle it?"), and that you respond to all these with **Empathy** (Singer M.).

   Conversely, you must seek an understanding of how the rest of the patient's life has affected or produced his/her symptoms.

6. **You can give a neurobiologic explanation to set the stage for biologic treatment of depression or anxiety.**

117

> **Dr.:** Mr. S., sometimes people feel bad for so long that their body chemistry changes. They don't sleep well, feel tired all the time, get forgetful, and can't even enjoy things any more. I wonder if anything like that has happened to you?

To explore the antecedents and consequences of the symptoms, focus on one episode and analyze it carefully. Ask your patient about when the symptoms were worse recently and walk through the episode. Find out not only the symptoms, but also what the patient was doing, who else was there, and what were his/her associated thoughts or feelings. Or your patient can keep a diary, rating the severity of symptoms on a 1 to 10 scale several times a day, along with ratings of stress and notes about activities, foods, thoughts, and feelings. Note that physical responses to stress can be delayed for hours and days. When you debrief the patient about the diary, ask him/her, "What did you notice from keeping the diary?" and then "Are there some specific parts you want to talk about?" The goal is to get your patient to become an astute observer of the antecedents (thoughts, feelings, interactions, circumstances) of symptoms and his/her own behaviors, thoughts, feelings, and interactions that come as a result of the symptoms.

It is reasonable to acknowledge and share your own uncertainty about the cause of the symptoms. You can accept information the patient brings, but try to keep your treatment focused on improving function.

7. **Manage difficult interactive styles.** The most problematic styles are suffering, hostility, and dependence. Some patients need to suffer in order to feel worthy of care and love. Before you can respond empathically to a patient who is suffering, you must understand the phenomenon of suffering and accept the doctor's role to ameliorate suffering. To many of us, indoctrinated with the model of acute curable illness, the very notion of suffering may be foreign. Some suffering patients actually seem satisfied when told that nothing can be done for them. Your task with such patients is to appreciate their burden of suffering.

> **Dr.:** Mr. S., I just don't know how you keep going despite your symptoms. Not many people would be able to put up with what you do.

The shame and loss of control that come with symptoms can make people angry. Paradoxically that anger may be directed at the very people trying to help. You may have to acknowledge that anger is a normal part of illness but can get in the way of care.

Dr.: Mr. S., I can see that you are really upset about this problem. Many people would be. And I want to help, but we need to be able to work together on this. If you stay angry with me, it makes it harder for me to be helpful. What do you think?

Pt.: Yeah, I do get angry when I think of how my life has been messed up and when I think of all the trouble I've had with doctors who don't even believe how I'm suffering. But you've been OK, doctor, and I shouldn't be mad at you.

Dr.: Great! How about if you tell me what the worst part of it is for you now?

Dependence grows in most illnesses. After all, illness requires that other people do things for the patient that he/she normally does. People often become both more dependent and more frustrated by that very dependence. Sometimes their dependence seems out of proportion to the duties of clinicians, and you may need to explain how you can best work to help them, defining your own boundaries and limits.

Dr.: Mr. S., I know that you need to discuss your bowels with me some more. I think that's a good idea. But I need to do it during my regular telephone hours. Can you wait until I call you then? I could get back to you tomorrow between 3:00 and 5:00 PM.

8. **Use tests, referrals, and medications cautiously.** Medications for symptoms should be given on a scheduled basis rather than as needed, to avoid rewarding the symptom by taking a pill. The medication should be given for a specified period of time, and its effectiveness should be judged on how well it improves the patient's function (going to work or class, going out, cooking or cleaning...) rather than on its ability to remove or reduce symptoms. If the medication doesn't improve function, it should be discontinued.

9. **Be careful what you call the problem.** Some wastebasket diagnoses, such as "viral syndrome" or "a little arthritis," can lead to needless worry and misconceptions. You can call protracted fatigue just that, not "the chronic fatigue syndrome." We suggest that you try to lead your patient to understand that emotional issues often amplify physical symptoms, especially fatigue, generalized aches and pains, and malaise. Another useful term, understandable to patients, is *heightened somatic aware-*

119

ness, a condition that may occur when brain chemistry changes, e.g., in depression or anxiety, and that may respond to medication for those disorders.

10. **Support, even applaud, your patient's efforts.**

> **Dr.:** Mr. S., knowing how tough all this is for you, I'm impressed with all you do manage to do. Getting up and getting dressed in the morning is sometimes something you can barely do, yet you do that and continue to work half time. That takes a great deal of grit and I admire you for it.

11. **Help your patient think about his/her situation from a different perspective.** Once you are convinced that no further workup will help at this time, don't keep taking the symptom history again and again. Instead, ask the patient what he/she has been able to do despite the symptoms. Explore with him/her what additional things he/she might do to keep active and feel better.

12. Help patients become aware of the negative things they say to themselves about the symptoms (e.g., "I guess I'll never be able to do that again.") and substitute new things ("I know I can do it if I take it slow"). Have patients schedule pleasurable events despite their symptoms and find new sources of self-esteem.

13. See the family. Get their perspective. Identify ways the patient's family and social system might be reinforcing the symptoms.

14. **Use mental health referrals** if you are unsure about the presence of a psychologic disorder or if your patient seems not to be making the progress you hoped for. Tell your patient that you would like to bring in a consultant to help both of you to find additional ways to improve coping with difficult symptoms. Be sure your patient understands that you will remain his/her doctor but that you need consultative help. Then choose a consultant with whom you can work closely. If you are working with an anonymous mental health system, insist that the consultant call you after a visit or two with your patient. Ask your patient to ask the consultant to do just that.

15. **Schedule regular visits**, more frequently than you or the patient might otherwise choose.

> **Dr.:** Mr. S., when should we see you next?
>
> *continued*

> **Pt.:** Oh, probably two months would be OK.
>
> **Dr.:** Gosh, that seems too far off. Let's make it about six weeks, OK?
>
> **Pt.:** Sure, Doc. Whatever you say.

Avoid telling the patient that he/she doesn't need to come back to see you unless he/she has a new problem. A new problem is inevitable. Scheduling regular visits decreases escalating symptoms and doctor-shopping. Regular visits disconnect the link between having the symptoms and seeing the doctor.

PITFALLS TO AVOID

1. Testing and referring until the patient stops coming, or telling the patient that there's nothing wrong and he/she need not come back.

2. Becoming impatient. Approaching this complex patient with a long history of complaints determined to cut through diagnostic uncertainty and solve the problem once and for all.

3. Measuring your success in terms of relieving or explaining the symptoms.

4. Responding to somatizing patients with feelings of anger, frustration, or hopelessness while remaining unaware of your own feelings.

5. Failing to recognize and respect the degree that your patient is suffering even though you find no organic cause.

PEARL

Focus on helping the somatizing patient keep or regain function, not on curing the disease.

SELECTED READINGS

Barsky AJ. A 37-year-old man with multiple somatic complaints. JAMA 1997;278:673–679.

Barsky AJ. Patients who amplify bodily sensations. Ann Intern Med 1979;91:63–70.

121

Cantor C. Phantom Illness. Boston: Houghton Mifflin, 1996.

Goldberg DP, Bridges K. Somatic presentations of psychiatric illness in primary care setting. J Psychosom Res 1988;32:137–144.

Gordon GH. Treating somatizing patients. West J Med 1987;147: 88–91.

Kaplan C, Lipkin M, Gordon GH. Somatization in primary care: patients with unexplained and vexing medical complaints. J Gen Intern Med 1988;3:178–190.

Kroenke K, Mangelsdorff AD. Common symptoms in ambulatory care: incidence, evaluation, therapy and outcome. Am J Med 1969; 86:262–266.

Peabody FW. The Care of the Patient. JAMA 1927;88:877 reprinted in Conn Med 1976;40:545–552.

Quill TE, Suchman AL. Uncertainty and control: learning to live with medicine's limitations. Humane Medicine. 1993;9:109–120.

Servan-Schreiber D. Coping effectively with patients who somatize. Woman's Health in Primary Care. 1998;1(5):435–447.

Smith RC. Somatization disorder: defining its role in clinical medicine. J Gen Intern Med 1991;6:168–175.

Taylor GJ, Bagby RM, Parker JDA. The alexithymia construct. Psychosomatics. 1991;32:153–164.

CHAPTER 20
Long-Term Suffering

PROBLEM

Patients with chronic symptoms of pain, fatigue, and malaise fall into two categories: those whose symptoms are associated with an identifiable causative organic disease such as osteoarthritis, and those with similar symptoms but no well-defined organic cause. Included in this last category are patients with problems such as fibromyalgia and persisting fatigue. Some of these patients demonstrate variants of somatization, and some have secondary psychologic symptoms, such as depression following years of fatigue or pain. Another way to divide this complex group of patients with long-term symptoms is between those who seem to develop illness behavior, becoming sick and disabled by their symptoms, and those who suffer the symptoms but remain functional, avoid seeking medical care, and do not view themselves as ill.

PRINCIPLES

1. Any symptom or condition that goes on more than six months has outcomes more dependent on psychosocial and behavioral characteristics than on biological characteristics.

2. Chronic pain, usually back, pelvis, head, and face, are common in the practice of medicine. They may or may not result in the patient becoming chronically ill.

3. Pain and fatigue interfere with all function.

4. **Treating a chronic condition demands different strategies than treating acute conditions.** Acute disorders may be curable. Chronic disorders probably are not, so doctor and patient must adjust their expectations accordingly. When working with chronic pain, we should focus on maintaining or improving the patient's function and accept that this task will continue indefinitely.

5. After the initial evaluation, the patient with chronic problems can take a lead role in carrying out treatment. Whereas in treating acute illness, the doctor directs the interventions, in treating chronic illness the patient does much of the treating work and the doctor coaches.

PROCEDURES

1. **Make sure that you and your patient agree that the diagnosis is a chronic disorder.** Patients may be reluctant to accept that there is no further testing or treatment, and may want to search for another diagnosis.

2. Acknowledge any differences in understanding and in diagnosis between you and the patient, and **try to find some common ground.** Use phrases such as, "Let's make sure I understand you ....," "Here's my perspective ....," or "You might even wonder if I am missing something or if I will be able to help."

3. **Find out the meaning of the pain or fatigue to the patient functionally, symbolically, and historically.** What can't the patient do because of this symptom? What does it tell him/her about himself/herself as a person? Who else had something like this? What happened to them?

4. **Set limits on yourself.** Define what you can do and what you can't do. For example, you can't make the symptom go away.

> **Pt.:** I just want the pain to go away.
>
> **Dr.:** And it must be very frustrating to you that I can't make the pain go away.

5. The goal of treatment with narcotics and other medications should be to improve function despite chronic symptoms. If this goal is not being met, the treatment is ineffective.

6. Remember that your patients with chronic symptoms are truly suffering, and you can let them know that you understand that. Acknowledging suffering validates the patient's condition and gives you a route of care: even if you can't lessen pain, you may help the patient's response to it.

7. Using the disability model, applaud your patient's accomplishments despite his/her problem.

8. If the patient requests disability, clarify your role. Is it to document findings, to provide clinical cure, to adjudicate a dispute, or to certify disability? Some roles are mutually incompatible.

9. Refer patients early to a chronic pain management program that emphasizes behavioral approaches.

Dr.: Ms. R., given the suffering you have, I'm impressed that you are able to function as well as you do, caring for yourself and shopping and all.

PITFALLS TO AVOID

1. Promising to get rid of the patient's chronic pain or persisting fatigue.

2. Failing to disabuse your thoroughly evaluated patient of the notion that he/she should continue to seek etiologic diagnoses.

3. Undertreating or overtreating pain with narcotics.

PEARL

Respect the chronicity of symptoms and the potential for improved function and self-esteem.

SELECTED READINGS

Blackwell B, Gutmann M. The management of chronic illness behavior. In: McHugh S, Ballis M, eds. Illness Behaviors. NY: Plenum, 1987.

Carey TS, Hadler NM. The role of the primary physician in disability determination for social security insurance and worker's compensation. Ann Intern Med 1986;104:706–710.

Cassel EJ. The nature of suffering and the goals of medicine. N Engl J Med 1982;306:639–645.

Dworkin SF. Illness behavior and dysfunction: review of concepts and applications to chronic pain. Can J Physiol Pharmacol 1991;69: 662–671.

Fordyce W. Pain and suffering—a reappraisal. Am Psychol 1988;43: 276–283.

Gureje O, Von Korff M, Simon GE, Gater R. Persistent pain and well being. JAMA 1998;280:147–151.

Iazonni LI. What should I say? Communication around disability. Ann Intern Med 1998;129:661–665.

Sullivan MD, Turner JA, Romano J. Chronic pain in primary care: identification and management of psychosocial factors. J Fam Pract 1991;32:193–199.

Vandereycken W, Meermann R. Chronic illness behavior and noncompliance with treatment: pathways to an interactional approach. Psychother Psychosom 1988;50:182–191.

Wooley SSC, Blackwell B, Winget C. A learning theory model of chronic illness behavior: theory, treatment, and research. Psychosom Med 1978;40:379–401.

CHAPTER 21

The Transition From Definitive Care to Palliative Care

PROBLEM

The move from definitive care to palliative care requires you to work on different tasks, including the patient's current concerns. Those concerns, shared by many patients as their disease progresses past the curable stages, include:

a) control of pain and other symptoms and body functions (eating, nausea, breathing, anxiety, constipation,...).

b) how to talk with spouses and children about the impact of this change.

c) how to find sources of personal support.

d) how to avoid side effects of medicines and fears of addiction.

e) life tasks still undone.

PRINCIPLES

1. When you have no more definitive treatments left to offer a patient, you still have your continuing help and concern to offer. You can assure the patient that you will not abandon him/her.

2. Doctors are part of the orchestration of a sick person's life, and you should plan to attend family conferences and contribute information about the patient's physical and emotional needs. These may be emotional encounters for both you and the family.

3. There's a lot to know about end-of-life health issues including pain management, family counseling, support groups, and home hospice. Mastering this information and knowing about resources for the terminally ill and their families is part of the job. The first step is often identifying a person in your community or institution who knows and coordinates these resources.

PROCEDURES

1. At first this resembles giving bad news again, only more so. **Use empathy as your primary tool.** Listen carefully for the patient's thoughts, feelings, and concerns. It also helps to anticipate what the patient must be going through.

Dr.: Shirley, this is going to be hard to hear. I'm afraid we don't have anything else we can use that fights the cancer specifically.

(pause)

Pt. (smiling): Oh, come on now, Doctor. That's what you said before, and then the specialists gave me those other treatments. What now? A bone marrow transplant? I'll do whatever I have to to lick this.

Dr.: I know you will. And I appreciate your energy and enthusiasm. That's why it's doubly hard for me to talk with you about this.

Pt.: I don't understand, Doctor. What are you saying?

Dr.: I'm saying that after talking with all the specialists we can't find anything more that will slow or stop the cancer. That means that we need to change gears and work on helping you to cope with this situation.

Pt. (scared): Oh my God, Doctor. You can't really mean this. You can't be serious. Doctor, I have kids in school—nobody else knows how to take care of them.

Dr.: I know this isn't what we planned for.

Pt. (crying): This isn't fair. Isn't there some treatment left?

Dr.: You're right. It isn't fair. And even though we can't hope for a cure, I imagine there's lots of other things that are important to you now that we need to work on.

Pt.: Oh my God! What am I going to do now?

Dr.: Well I still want to be your doctor. What do we need to do today, right now, about this?

Pt.: I don't even know what to tell Dave or the kids.

Dr.: Why not bring them in tomorrow and we can talk about it. There is a social worker who works with cancer patients who can help us talk about it together.

The patient will need to modify his/her goals, and may need to begin a long parting process from family, friends, and his/her life. The patient may suffer loneliness and fears, and will need people to talk with about those feelings. Your task now is to help the patient through this difficult process.

2. **Don't rush. Stay there.** Don't shy away from the patient's feelings of anger, regret, or sadness. Don't shy away from discussing the patient's hopes, desires, and goals. Ask about specific fears and concerns, and be willing to address them.

3. **Take time to grieve yourself.**

4. Make sure you, too, are able to make the transition to palliative care. Become familiar with the principles of palliative care and symptom management.

5. **Check to be sure that your patient's values are honored** during his/her terminal care. If the patient is part of a large and active family, see that family visits are accommodated and keep designated family members well informed. Be sure that your patient has access to spiritual advisors and has an advocate for his/her needs.

PITFALLS TO AVOID

1. Abandoning the patient when your curative therapy reaches its endpoint.

2. Failing to give up curative therapy long after its effectiveness has ceased.

3. Running away from grief.

4. Failing to empathize with the patient's great loss or with grieving relatives.

5. Becoming angry when the brave patient who bore pain nobly deteriorates into dependence.

PEARL

Make sure that the patient knows that you will stay with him/her, that you are in it for the long haul.

SELECTED READINGS

Doyle D, Hanks GWC, MacDonald N. (edit.) Oxford textbook of palliative medicine. 2nd ed. Oxford: Oxford U. Press, 1998.

Kjaer M. The therapy of cancer pain and its integration into a comprehensive supportive case strategy. Ann Oncol 1997;8:515–9.

Levenson SA. Subacute and transition care handbook: defining, delivering and improving care. St. Louis:1996, Crucam Pub.

O'Boyle CA, Waldron D. Quality of life issues in palliative medicine. J Neurol 1997;244(supp4):S18–25.

Seely JF, Scott JF, Mount BM. The need for specialized training programs in palliative medicine. Can Med Assoc J 1997;157: 1395–1397.

Stiefel F, Guex P. Palliative and supportive care: at the frontier of medical omnipotence. Ann Oncol 1997;7:135–138.

Weissman DE. Consultation in palliative medicine. Arch Intern Med 1997;157:733–737.

CHAPTER 22

End-of-Life Discussions

PROBLEM

End-of-life discussions must take place in both longstanding and new doctor–patient relationships. We need to know our patients' preferences and to reach plans that feel right to them and seem possible to us.

PRINCIPLES

1. End-of-life discussions are a part of every patient's long-term care. You can begin the discussion when the patient is feeling healthy and has the chance to think about his/her choices and to talk with his/her family.

2. The doctor can talk about end-of-life issues with the same forthright, frank attitude used toward other health topics.

3. **Our own feelings may make it hard to converse about death.** We may avoid discussing dying and death if it contrasts too harshly with our wish to bring hope and healing. If we have had a long-term relationship with the patient we may be suffering from guilt, sadness, or fears about his/her demise. If we are just now meeting the patient, we may feel annoyed that such discussions haven't been held earlier by the patient's primary doctor. We may fear seeming too blunt and unfeeling if we broach subjects as painful as death or resuscitation plans with a patient who hardly knows us. We don't like to upset people or worry them unnecessarily. Indeed, we need to find a way to bring up the subject without alarming or frightening our patient. In most cases, however, the patient is comforted by an open discussion of these issues.

4. It is key to understand how your patient's values drive his/her specific requests.

5. There are two sorts of advance directives, **living wills**—of limited applicability—and the more useful **appointment of another person as a legal representative for health care decisions.** Both take effect only when the patient loses decision-making capacity; neither requires a lawyer to complete, and both can be purchased wherever legal documents are sold (such as at stationery stores).

6. The Patient Self-Determination Act, a Federal law, requires that every health care organization receiving federal funds have a sys-

tem in place for asking patients on admission if they have advance directives, and for providing information if they don't.

7. Policies and laws dictate who can represent a patient who has no decision-making capacity and no advance directives.

PROCEDURES

1. The sequence is:
   a) Bring up the topic.
   b) Ask what ideas and experiences the patient has about advance directives (perhaps from family, friends, or the media).
   c) Ask who else might be available to speak for the patient if he/she is not able to communicate.
   d) Make the discussion formal. Ask the patient to complete documents appointing that person as a legal health-care representative if he/she is unable to speak for himself/herself.
   e) Ask that person to document acceptance of this role.
   f) Rediscuss it all in the future; offer to include others in the discussion if the patient desires.

2. Most hospitals and other care facilities have policies that ask us to determine resuscitation plans and limitations for all our admitted patients. That gives us a good excuse and a good starting point for discussion of the patient's wishes.

Dr.: Mrs. A?

Pt.: Yes?

Dr.: We have discussed a plan for your care here in the hospital, but sometimes things happen that we don't anticipate. One of the areas we always ask about, and I think it is a good idea, is this: If something should happen to you where you weren't able to plan your treatment with me, what would you want us to do? For example, are there any conditions under which you would or would not like certain kinds of medical care?

Pt.: Like what, doctor?

continued

Dr.: Well, let's take the worst case scenario. Suppose your heart stopped or you stopped breathing. If that should happen, it's unlikely that we could return you to your present state.

Pt.: I see.

Dr.: Now some people value life at all costs. Others would not want to be in certain conditions permanently, for example, needing a machine in order to breathe or being unable to communicate.

Pt.: Well, I wouldn't want that. If that happens and I can't get better, just stop the treatment and let me go.

Dr.: OK, I understand. I can certainly honor that wish. Of course that doesn't mean we would not try hard to keep you alive and functioning well up to that time.

Pt.: I don't want to be stuck on any machines.

Dr.: I see. You know, this discussion really has bearing only if you are unable to communicate with us. As long as you can tell us what you want, we will try to do just that. We're only talking about what you would want done if you couldn't tell us at the time we needed to make a decision, like if you were unconscious or too sick to understand what's wrong or what the treatment choices are.

Pt.: I understand. That's fine, Doctor. I don't want to be in pain and I don't want to be dependent on others for my care. I'm mostly concerned about being dependent.

Dr.: I can imagine. That's a common concern, and I can surely understand it. What does "dependent" mean for you?

The doctor attempts to learn more about his patient and present the patient with what the end-of-life decisions are.

These conversations should be well documented and the documents, along with more formal election of a health care representative, should be kept in a safe place; but it is important that copies be given to the patient's doctor and important relatives and representatives.

Be sure that your patient is cognitively and emotionally capable of making these decisions before beginning this discussion: He/she can describe what is or could be wrong, understands the nature of proposed treatments and likely outcomes, can compare the value of different options, and can indicate a preference.

3. **Ask all your patients about their desires for resuscitation**, even if they're young. Document all these discussions in the pa-

tient's chart. Note exactly what the patient was asked and what his/her answers were.

4. Even though patients come to you already having filled out some forms about their desires in case of death or inability to communicate, you still have to have a conversation about end-of-life issues.

5. **Be sure that the key family members understand your patient's wishes.** Often times they have been left out of the conversation and are surprised, perhaps disbelieving when you cite your patient's desires. Ask who key members are and whether they know your patient's wishes.

PITFALLS TO AVOID

1. Shying away from discussions about dying and death. Hoping that you aren't on call when the patient dies.

2. Failing to document end-of-life discussions with the patient.

3. Leaving key players out of the discussion, chancing explosive conflicts among relatives at big decision points.

PEARL

Discuss end-of-life issues regardless of the patient's age, and document your conversation.

SELECTED READINGS

Carney MT, Morrison RS. Advance directives: when, why, and how to start talking. Geriatrics. 1997;52:65–6, 69–74.

Doukas DH, McCullough LB. The values history: the evaluation of the patient's values and advance directives. J Fam Pract 1991;32: 145–153.

Finger AL. Enlisting a patient's adult children as allies. Medical Economics 1997;74(3):173–189.

Gordon GH, Dunn P. Advance directives and the patient self-determination act. Hosp Pract 1992;27:39–42.

Hofmann JC et al. Patient preferences for communication with physicians about end-of-life decisions. Ann Intern Med 1997;127:1–12.

Johnston SC, Pfeifer MP. Patient and physician roles in end-of-life decision making. J Gen Intern Med. 1998;13:43–45.

Lynn J, Miles SH, Olick R. Making living wills and health care proxies more useful. Patient Care 1998;32(9):181–192.

Sulmasy DP et al. The accuracy of substituted judgments in patients with terminal diagnoses. Ann Intern Med 1998;128:621–629.

Teno JM, Stevens M, Spernak S, Lynn J. Role of written advance directives in decision making. J Gen Intern Med 1998;13:439–446.

Tulsky JA, Fischer GS, Rose MR, Arnold RM. Opening the black box: how do physicians communicate about advance directives? Ann Intern Med 1998;129:441–449.

Uhlmann RF, Pearlman RA, Cain KC. Physicians' and spouses' predictions of elderly patients' resuscitation preferences. J Gerontol 1998;43:M115–121.

CHAPTER 23
Talking With the Family

PROBLEM

Meetings with large family groups can be difficult. Most meetings have a central focus, usually about the health of one of its members. The meeting itself may be chaotic and challenging. What should happen at family meetings? What is your role?

Case Study

Mr. A., a retired engineer with chronic obstructive pulmonary disease, fell and fractured five ribs, developing a pneumothorax. Mr. A. had been firm about his desire for "no heroics." But because of the pneumothorax, in rapid succession he endured placement of two chest tubes; a move to the ICU; and (as his oxygenation fell) an endotracheal tube, in conjunction with which he was put on a respirator. By then he was unconscious and unable to communicate. Three days later, family members asked to come to talk to the doctors involved in his care.

In an ICU conference room are four adult children, two in-laws, one chaplain, an intern, the attending physician, and a nurse manager. The medical team had previously met together to discuss care on several occasions. They were uncertain about his prognosis and concerned that they had already done more than the patient would have wanted. No major divisions had appeared between the caretakers. Prior to the family meeting, the caretaking staff wondered what to tell the family and what questions to address.

What should happen at this meeting?

PRINCIPLES

1. **Identifying participants by name and role shows respect for the family and helps you locate the key decision-makers.**

2. To make sure that everyone shares the same understanding, it helps to briefly summarize the biomedical facts of the case and any decisions that need to be made.

3. If the patient has decision-making capacity, you should represent the patient. If not, be sure that the family understands that you need their help in representing the patient, not in making *their*

decisions for him/her. Know the laws governing who can legally represent the patient if he/she hasn't completed an advance directive.

4. The urgency of family decision making will vary greatly from situation to situation.

5. The physician can use the same techniques in the family conference as in the medical interview, eliciting a complete agenda, assessing what the family understands about the situation and what ideas they have about what can be done and what the doctor should do. As in the medical interview, the doctor should listen carefully to all the involved parties before giving an extensive explanation.

6. It is important to clear up any divisions in the medical team before involving the family. Make sure that you understand the perspective of everyone on the health care team. Do all parties share the same assumptions and goals?

7. Whenever any two family members are gathered in times of crisis, there is likely to be conflict. Some members may have come from afar, they may have different values and opinions, and long-standing rifts in the family may surface when members are asked to take control of decisions. The physician does not want to become ensnared in feuds or power struggles.

PROCEDURES

1. Get your facts and probabilities straight before the meeting. **Don't leave your responses to chance.** The family will be using the information from this conference to make decisions, and if you have recommendations you will want to support them with facts.

2. **Establish identities and roles.** Explain the need to know who everyone is and perform introductions. "I know you will have a lot of questions for us; but before we begin, we all need to know each other's names and our exact relationship to Mr. A."

3. **Identify the family spokesperson and anyone with a special legal position**, such as power of attorney for health care. "I need to ask you a couple of technical questions. Have you in any way designated a single spokesperson for most of our communication? If not, it would be helpful if the family could confer and let us know who that will be. Has Mr. A. chosen and designated any

of you to have power of attorney for health care? Does he have a living will?"

You can ask that the family identify a spokesperson for future communication and ask them to focus on this discussion: Which family member is most comfortable with these issues? In emergencies, whom do you want us to call first?

4. After these introductory clarifications, you are ready to discuss family concerns. "OK. I think we're ready to begin. I could start by summarizing the medical situation, and then I'd like to hear your concerns and questions." Then, hearing the family members' questions, rephrase them to ensure understanding and to focus on values and goals.

5. By the end of the meeting, you and your patient's family should have some common understandings about your patient's status and your agreed-on plans. It helps to reiterate them now.

> **Dr.:** Let me see if I can restate what we're agreed on. John is still on the ventilator but he had wished to avoid such a treatment, and we're agreed that we should stop our efforts if he's no better in two days. We all find that a tough decision but think it fits best with John's wishes. Is that where we're all at?

6. If the family is in conflict, restate and clarify the positions of those in conflict. Then ask if these conflicts have happened before and how they were resolved. Finally ask if the family would like help resolving it now and identify resources that might help.

PITFALLS TO AVOID

1. Coming to the family conference without a plan.

2. Coming to the family conference without adequate information about the patient.

3. Talking too much, listening and hearing too little.

4. Failing to identify the family decision-makers and the patient's legal spokesperson.

5. Failing to emphasize patient autonomy and your efforts to do what the patient would have been telling you to do if he/she were able to communicate.

6. Failing to describe the patient's situation and possible outcomes accurately.

PEARL

Seek a shared understanding of the medical situation and what the patient would have wanted.

SELECTED READINGS

Campbell TL, McDaniel SH. Conducting a family interview. In: Lipkin M, Putnam SM, Lazare A, eds. The medical interview. clinical care, education and research. NY: Springer-Verlag, 1995;15: 178–186.

Erstling SS, Devlin J. The single-session family interview. J Fam Pract 1989;28:556–560.

Hahn SR, Ferner JS, Bellin EH. The doctor–patient–family relationship: a compensatory alliance. Ann Intern Med 1988:109:884–889.

Mulhern RK, Crisco JJ, Camitta BM. Patterns of communication among pediatric patients with leukemia, parents, and physicians: prognostic disagreements and misunderstandings. J Pediatr 1991; 99:480–483.

CHAPTER 24
Being With a Dying Patient

PROBLEM

Once it is clear that your patient is dying, it may seem to you that your work is done and that you would be better off elsewhere. If your view of death is that it is a defeat in your battle, you may want to retire from the front. But you still have work to do. Over 80% of deaths in the United States occur in health care institutions, and thus in the hands of medical professionals. We have taken over the family's tasks and are puzzled about what to do.

Case Study

Mr. A., an 83-year-old man suffering from dementia, fell in his nursing home and fractured his hip. He was operated on and is now four days postoperative, being treated with anticoagulants and his usual cardiac medications. He also has severe mitral insufficiency and heart failure. This morning he was seen to vomit several times and perhaps to aspirate, and has become tachypneic, hypoxic, and restless. His chest x-ray shows diffuse infiltrates suggestive of heart failure and a very large heart. Oxygen and diuretic therapy seem to make little difference, and he has progressively deteriorated over the day. When the on-call doctor came to see him at 11:00 PM, the patient was hypotensive, comatose, and diaphoretic, and the doctor thought he was moribund. He asked the nurse to call Mrs. A. She was on her way in to the hospital.

What should the doctor plan to do now? What do we do for dying patients?

PRINCIPLES

1. We must attempt to ensure the patient's comfort, even if at the cost of shortening life somewhat. Dying need not be suffering.

2. Your main focus must extend to the family and friends of the dying patient. They need comfort, support, and clear evidence that their loved one is not suffering.

We remember this brief dialogue:

> **Dr.: (leaning over the bed to talk to a frail, terminally ill patient):** Ruth, is there anything at all that I can do for you?

continued

Pt.: (faintly) Well, I would like just a few fried oysters.

The doctor mobilized the resources: he called a hospital dietitian, who called a local seafood restaurant, who delivered a special plate. The patient ate and appreciated the oysters. The next day the doctor leaned over her bed and asked the same question.

Pt.: (still more faint) Well, perhaps just one small piece of sweet potato pie.

PROCEDURES

1. **Be available. If possible, be on the scene to orchestrate events at the deathbed.** If you are unable to sit with the dying person, advocate for a hospital staff person to be present or closely available. With Mr. A., the doctor arrived ahead of the patient's family and arranged for a nursing staff person to sit with the dying patient and his family even after the doctor left. He made sure that the patient's room and bedclothes were tidy, and used small doses of intravenous morphine to make the patient comfortable. Then he simply sat at the bedside.

2. **Just be there.** The hardest action for many of us is no action, just being present. We have to recognize that being there is a real activity that requires effort. Stay there while the family expresses their grief. Be prepared for emotional and loud expressions of grief, along with some surprises. If you are expecting tears, you may instead encounter fear, anger, or confusion. Loss affects people in many different ways.

3. **Consider the family members as your new patients.** Focus especially on the intimates—parent, spouse, caretaker. They will usually be identifiable because they'll be central in place and action; but if you don't know who they are, ask. Introduce yourself again and be sure that you note their names and their relationship to the dying patient.

4. **Practice empathy by asking how the family members are feeling.** You can support them by expressing understanding.

5. **Ask to hear about the patient's life.** Who was this person for them? What sort of a person was he?

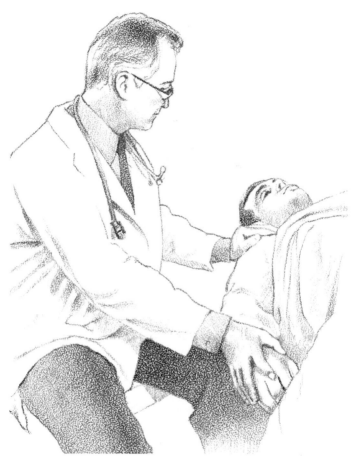

Being with a Dying Patient

Dr.: Mrs. A., I never had much of a chance to get to know Mr. A. Can you tell me what sort of a person he was?

Other good questions include: "How did you two meet?" "How long have you two been together?" The more the grieving relatives talk about the dying person, the calmer and more soothed they will be.

6. If you knew this patient enough to add to the narrative, you can add your comments, especially positive ones.

> **Dr.:** You know, I never met Mr. A. before today and when I saw him this morning he was pretty confused, but I had the feeling that he must have been a kind person.
>
> **Mrs. A.:** That's him exactly. He always was kind to me.

7. If the patient is a potential organ donor, ask if he/she had ever said anything to the family about organ donation. Did the patient ever indicate that he/she would want parts of his/her body to help others? Did the patient indicate it on his/her driver's license? If so, you can call the appropriate staff to talk with the family about the process of donation. Be able to discuss "what happens next," such as who will call the funeral home.

8. If you were present at the death, you might want to consider some sort of follow-up action, such as sending a card or even attending the funeral.

PITFALLS TO AVOID

1. Leaving arrangements and communication with the family to the nurse.

2. Avoiding anything personal. Talking with the family about biomedical and technical issues.

> **Dr.:** His myocardium simply could not maintain an adequate cardiac output. We tried diuresis and unloading therapy.

3. Missing the chance to hear the family's feelings and memories.

PEARL

Sometimes just showing up says more than words.

SELECTED READINGS

Irvine P. The attending at the funeral. New Eng J Med 1985; 1704–1705.

Lynn J, Teno JM, Phillips RS, Wu AW, Desbiens N, Harold J, Claessens MT, Wenger N, Kreling B, Connors AF Jr. Perceptions by family members of the dying experience of older and seriously ill patients. Study to understand prognoses and preferences for outcomes and risks of treatments. *Ann Intern Med* 1997;126:97–106.

Steinmetz D, Walsh M, Gabel LL, Williams PT. Family physicians' involvement with dying patients and their families. Attitudes, difficulties, and strategies. Arch Fam Med 1993;2:753–760.

Tolle S, Elliot DL, Girard DE. How to manage patient death and care for the bereaved. Postgrad Med 1985;78(2):87–92.

Tolle SW, Elliot DC, Hickam DH. Physician attitudes and practices at the time of patient deaths. Arch Intern Med 1984;144:2389–2391.

Part V
Behavioral Health Risks

Part

Behavioral Health Risks

CHAPTER 25
Assessing Risk Behaviors

PROBLEM

It is essential to obtain accurate data about the patient's current health-maintenance activity, as well as an accurate **risk history.** Our efforts encounter a huge number of social and personal issues that these questions encompass. How do you direct your inquiry to learn what you need to know about the patient's current behavior? What do you need to know?

PRINCIPLES

1. It helps to **distinguish a true social history** (i.e., information about the patient's family, interests, and social milieu) **from a medical risk history about behaviors** (like smoking, drinking, and risky activities). These latter items are clearly NOT part of a social history and belong in a different section of the interview, an area we call *HEALTH BEHAVIOR AND HEALTH RISKS.*

2. As always, no checklist is as good as careful listening and the ability to follow where our patients lead us. We do best with an open-ended inquiry, asking our patients to tell us about their concerns, using a lot of "what else?" questions, and staying out of their way.

3. The interviewer must be aware that **people are sensitive,** and these discussions about risk are the place for the interviewer's most **gentle, nonjudgmental technique.** You may need to preface some questions with an explanation: "These are questions I ask all my patients," or "In order to understand your health risks, I have to inquire about some areas that you usually keep private. I need the information to do a complete and thorough job here."

4. Precision is hard to come by in these areas. Patients will tell you that they exercise "quite a lot" or smoke "not that much." You'll have to help them be more exact. The task may not be easy.

> **Dr.:** "There are 20 cigarettes in a pack. How many cigarettes do you smoke a day?"
>
> **Pt.:** Oh, some days I don't hardly smoke at all. Maybe in the evening.

PROCEDURES

1. **Establish a section of your database that includes health-maintenance behaviors and health-risk behaviors.** A checklist is a good way to begin and to document the discussion, but then you need to discuss the list with your patient, learning how he/she views the importance of all the components. Begin your discussion by signposting: "We are going to concern ourselves with things that you do that help you stay healthy and then with things you do that endanger your health."

2. At the onset, outline for your patient the three main categories of behavior you want to inquire into: **prevention, health promotion, and finally risk assessment.** Prevention includes immunizations, safety procedures, wearing seat belts, and practicing safe sex. Health promotion includes diet, exercise, and medical screening procedures.

3. **Ask about the entire gamut of drugs:** toxic chemicals, alcohol, cigarettes, other tobacco products, street drugs (cocaine, heroin, etc.), prescribed drugs, over-the-counter medications, and health-food-store drugs. Most patients don't understand that these and even certain prescribed medications, such as birth control pills, are really drugs. Some will tell you that herbal remedies are "natural," and therefore don't have the same potential for harm as synthetic compounds. It is always useful to ask the patient if he/she is taking, injecting, or ingesting anything that might have any sort of side effects or potential for damage.

4. **Ask the patient about risky behavior:** driving cars without high seat backs or seat belts, riding a motorcycle without a helmet, skydiving, mountain climbing .... Ask if the patient keeps guns at home and how he/she stores them. In addition to asking the patient, "Do you do any risky sporting or recreational activities," ask about risky sexual behavior: multiple sexual partners or sex without condoms.

5. **Ask about other dangerous situations such as community or domestic violence.** It is estimated that half of all women will suffer some kind of assault by an intimate. The leading cause of death for young men is murder. Ask, "Are you currently living in fear of violence from anyone?" If the answer is "yes," you need to have referral resources for your patients. You also need to know the state and municipal laws regarding your duty to report evidence of injury. Doctors have a role in detecting and decreasing violence by talking to the potential perpetrators of violence.

Ask about anger. "How do you handle anger?" "Do you ever get in trouble when you are angry? Hurt someone? Get in fights? Get arrested?" Ask these questions of all patients: male or female; heterosexual or homosexual; young, middle-aged, or elderly. To learn about our patient's risk of violent injury, we must ask.

6. When you and your patient identify a behavior that he/she wants to change, you can **begin to enlist your patient in the change process.** Begin with staging, then adapt your behavior to your patient's current stage (see Chapter 16).

PITFALLS TO AVOID

1. Mixing up social history (who this person is, what his/her life is about, who else is important to the patient, etc.) with health hazards and health behavior. It is an error to assume that you are acquiring a social history when you are looking into health behavior or vice versa.

2. Assuming that you have so many questions to ask that you need to cut the patient off from expressing his/her concerns.

3. Becoming overwhelmed by the extent of the problem so that you avoid the entire issue of healthy and unhealthy behavior.

4. Getting in arguments with your patient about what is "safe" and what is "risky."

Dr.: Tell me what you do to stay healthy.

Pt.: Well, I get rolfed regularly. Then I take lots of vitamins, minerals, and herbs that I get at the Herb Cottage.

Dr.: That's a bunch of hogwash.

Pt.: Oh yeah? Says who?

Dr.: I do.

Pt.: Well, I just happen to have brought in some back issues of *Prevention Magazine* that I want you to read. They explain how you doctors never learned anything about nutrition, for example.

PEARL

Ask your patient about behavior, healthy and risky, and about the safety of his/her environment.

SELECTED READINGS

Cohen Cole SA. Difficult interviews: life style and life circumstance problems. In: The medical interview: the three function approach. St. Louis: Mosby, 1991:134–145.

Fillit HM, Hill J, Picarielle G, Warburton S. How the principles of geriatric assessment are shaping managed care. Geriatrics 1998;53: 76–89.

Gordon GH, Hickam DH. Talking with patients about screening. J Clin Outcomes Management 1998; 4:50–51.

Platt FW. The database. In: Conversation repair: case studies in doctor–patient communication. Boston: Little, Brown, 1995:117–138.

Prothrow-Stith D. Deadly consequences: how violence is destroying our teenage population and a plan to begin solving the problem. NY: Harper, 1993.

Smith RC. The medical record: health issues. In: The patient's story. Boston: Little, Brown, 1995:182–183.

CHAPTER 26
Nonadherence

PROBLEM

Patients disregard our recommendations far more often than we think. Data show that average adherence to prescribed medications varies from 30% to 70%. When we advise behavior changes such as cessation of smoking or drinking, we are far less successful.

Case Study

Ms. H. was admitted to the hospital last month for diabetic ketoacidosis. She had the worst numbers you have ever seen (blood sugar 880mG/dL, pH 7.1) and was comatose and hypotensive. After seven days in the intensive care unit she walked out, beaming, thanking everyone, and promising to bring in a crate of tamales for all. She had been well instructed in how to avoid future attacks of ketoacidosis.

Today, in the emergency department, you meet her again. Once again she is comatose, acidotic, hypovolemic, hyperglycemic, and ketotic. Her sister says that your patient hasn't been following her diet or taking her medications. One of your colleagues in the emergency department says that he, too, cared for her during a prior admission for ketoacidosis and that she is "simply noncompliant."

PRINCIPLES

1. **Our goal for patients is that they comply with our recommendations.** When they don't we label them as noncompliant. But adherence to doctors' orders may not be what we should expect. Patients may be adhering to their own beliefs about treatment and their own values concerning quality of life. The physician's concept of compliance is sometimes in conflict with the patient's values and the patient's determination to make his/her own decisions.

   The cost of noncompliance or nonadherence is currently estimated at $100 billion a year in the United States.

2. **No marker (social, racial, socioeconomic, educational, or other definable patient characteristic) predicts adherence or nonadherence.**

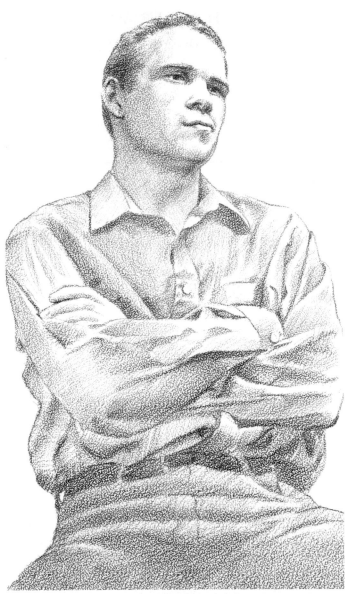

Noncompliance

3. **The best predictor of patient adherence so far determined is the doctor–patient relationship itself.**

   Factors leading to noncompliance include:
   a) physician failure to explain well.
   b) patient failure to understand the explanation.
   c) written material that is confusing or beyond the patient's reading skill level.
   d) cost of treatment in time, money, comfort, or effort.
   e) concern over troublesome or dangerous side effects.
   f) patient's lack of belief that the physician's recommendation will be helpful.
   g) conflict between patient's and physician's ideas of illness and therapies.
   h) conflict between patient's family and life context and doctor's therapeutic plans.
   i) patient fatigue or forgetfulness.

PROCEDURES

1. You must understand your patient's explanatory model of the illness, including his/her view of the diagnosis, its cause, and the appropriate treatment. Ask: "What did you think was the cause of your trouble? What sort of diagnoses have you been considering? What did you think we might best do?"

> **Dr. X.:** Well, Mr. Fine, before we go further, could you tell me what you thought this trouble was? What sort of diagnoses have you been considering?
>
> **Pt.:** What? You want to know what I think? I'm no doctor!
>
> **Dr. X.:** Sure, but I imagine that you had come up with a possible explanation or two for this trouble.
>
> **Pt.:** Well, actually I thought it might be some sort of infection, maybe in my sinuses.
>
> **Dr. X.:** I see, some sort of sinus infection. And what did you think we might best do for it?
>
> **Pt.:** Well, I figured some sort of antibiotic might fix it up.

Once in a while you will find your patient hesitant to tell you his/her theories. You can coax the patient.

Pt.: I don't know, Doc. I had no idea. That's why I came to you.

Dr. X.: Well, OK. But if you did know, what would it be?

Pt.: Oh, some sort of infection, maybe.

If you discover that your patient's ideas come close to your own, you should stress that agreement. Give the patient some praise for a good diagnosis or a good therapeutic plan.

Dr. X.: Sinus infection? Yes, I think you're right! You'll be opening up your own practice one of these days! I'm concerned with your lungs too. I think the infection may be in your sinuses and in your breathing tubes, your bronchi. I'd add bronchitis to the sinusitis diagnosis.

Pt.: I see. Worse yet, huh?

When you and your patient differ about this explanatory model, you must bring this disagreement to the surface and discuss it.

Dr.: Ms H., I have the feeling that we have different viewpoints about your diabetes and that we have different ideas about what should be done about it.

Pt.: What do you mean, Doctor?

Dr.: Well, my picture is that you have a chemical problem that you can only control by watching what you eat, sticking to the diet we've outlined, and taking insulin. If I hear you right, you think that now you are feeling better, you can go back to eating pretty much what you usually eat and that you don't need insulin unless you're sick enough to come into the hospital.

Pt.: I just don't know where I would get food like you want me to eat, Doctor. And my mother did fine without insulin for her diabetes.

Only when we've uncovered the conflict between the patient's understanding of the illness and the doctor's, can we expect to start trying to reach a treatment plan by negotiating with our patient.

2. **Ask your patient for his/her ideas about your plan.** What are the patient's tastes, habits, and limitations that will interfere with

his/her following it? Try to address these, asking his/her help in finding healthful alternatives where possible. Then, on return visits, ask how the customized plan is working and make adjustments with the patient's help. Always assume that the patient did not follow the plan perfectly. Then you may be able to alter it, making adherence easier.

Dr.: Mr. G., how have you been doing with the blood pressure medicines?

Pt.: Fine, Doc. OK.

Dr.: Well, none of us ever takes every pill we're supposed to take. We all miss some. How often do you miss them?

Pt.: Oh, hardly any. Maybe the evening pill; that's hard to remember sometimes.

Dr.: So how often?

Pt.: Oh, maybe one or two a week.

Dr.: You miss one or two a week?

Pt.: No, Doc, I only take one or two a week. But the morning pills I get most of the time. I only miss a couple.

Here is a treatment plan that we need to take back to the drawing board. Ask the patient for suggestions for helping him remember the blood pressure pills.

3. **Keep in contact with your patient.** When the patient has a serious illness, don't just send him/her home with directions for a return visit in a month. Call or have a staff person call periodically to check in by telephone.

4. **Voice your personal concern** for the patient's best possible outcome. "I'm concerned that you do what's needed to get well."

5. **Be sure that the patient understands.** Ask him/her to restate his/her plan.

6. **Do anticipatory problem solving.** "What might get in your way as you try to follow this plan?"

7. **Describe the potential side effects.** This will lead to more patients reporting having those side effects but fewer quitting the therapy because of the side effects.

PITFALLS TO AVOID

1. Believing that your job is to tell the patient what to do and that their job is to say, "OK, Doctor" and to do what you say.

2. Believing that your job is simply to fill patient requests and satisfy them.

3. Failing to determine the patient's ideas about diagnosis, causation, and therapy for the illness.

4. Failing to ask about potential barriers to adherence. On follow-up visits simply assuming that your patient is doing everything you had told him/her to do.

5. Spending a lot of money on hospital care and little on follow-up care.

6. Blaming the patient. Calling the patient noncompliant.

7. Trying to fix too many problems at one time.

PEARL

Attendance does not equal adherence. Work as hard to enlist your patient in his/her own care as you do in searching for the correct diagnosis and treatment.

SELECTED READINGS

Becker MH. Patient adherence to prescribed therapies. Med Care 1985;23:539–555.

Berg JS, Dischler J, Wagner DJ, Rara JJ, Palmer-Shelvin N. Medication compliance: a health care problem. Ann Pharmacother 1993;27:S3–S22.

Buckalow LW, Sallis RE. Patient compliance and medication perception. J Clin Psychol 1986;41:49–53.

Donovan JL, Blake DR. Patient non-compliance or reasoned decision-making? Soc Sci Med 1992;34:507–513.

Lazare A. The interview as a clinical negotiation. In: Lipkin M, Putnam SM, Lazare A, eds. The medical interview: clinical care, education and research. NY: Springer-Verlag, 1995:50–64.

McDermott MM, Schmitt B, Wallner E. Impact of medication nonadherence on coronary heart disease outcomes: a critical review. Arch Intern Med 1997;157:1921–1929.

Meichenbaum D, Turk DC. Facilitating treatment adherence: a practitioner's guidebook. NY: Plenum Press, 1987.

Quill TE, Brody H. Physician recommendations and patient autonomy: finding a balance between physician power and patient choice. Ann Intern Med 1996;125:763–769.

Scofield GR. The problem of (non-) compliance: is it patients or patience? HEC Forum. 1995;7:150–165.

Simpson MA, Buchman R, Stewart M, Maguire P, Lipkin M, Novack D. Doctor–patient communication: the Toronto consensus statement. BMJ 1991;303:1385–1387.

CHAPTER 27
Violence

PROBLEM

As a preventable cause of death and disability, violence is a significant risk. Screening for it is an important part of the physician's assessment. Violence is the leading cause of death in young American men. Sexual assault and domestic violence are common sources of injury in women. Other medical consequences of violence include post traumatic stress disorder, chronic pain, and sexual difficulties. We have to ask about the patient's management of anger and risk of violence, areas often left unexplored by physicians.

PRINCIPLES

1. Men and women ages 18 to 36 are most at risk of being victims of violence: men from strangers or acquaintances, women from intimates. Many people of both genders are victimized by verbal or emotional violence. This may affect the patient's attitude toward health and self-care.

2. The physician plays an important role in identifying and referring perpetrators of violence and patients who cannot manage their anger.

3. The doctor can provide some help for both community violence and domestic violence, once they are identified as part of the patient's risk assessment.

PROCEDURES

1. **Ask the key question, "Are you living in fear of violence from anyone?"** You can ask if your patient has been hurt by anyone else recently or in the past. Consider domestic violence, street and neighborhood violence, gang warfare, even road rage. If you see evidence of injury (broken bones, unexplained bruises, etc.) you should gently and kindly inquire about the source of those injuries, documenting the injuries and the patient's explanation for them in the chart.

2. **Remember that alcohol and drugs are often coproblems with violence.** If you find that the patient is a regular drinker or drug user, be sure to ask about fights and arguments.

3. **Ask all your patients who have a spouse or significant other what they do when disputes arise.** How do they settle them?

> **Dr.:** I know married life isn't always easy. What happens in your family when you and your spouse disagree?
>
> **Pt.:** Well, sometimes things get heated.
>
> **Dr.:** Heated?
>
> **Pt.:** Yeah, you know, angry.
>
> **Dr.:** What happens then?

4. **Ask if the patient or anyone else in the family ever had to go to the doctor because of an injury incurred at someone else's hand.**

5. **It is equally important to ask if the patient ever perpetrates violence.** Don't show gender bias when asking about the patient's use of violence. Both men and women use physical force to coerce or punish, but men's use of force more frequently results in injuries.

6. Ask about weapons and firearms in the home and what safeguards prevent their unintentional use.

> **Dr.:** When you get angry, what happens? (pause) Ever get in fights? (pause) Ever hurt anyone when you were angry? (pause) Ever have the police called because of something you did when you were angry? (pause)

   Note the pauses. As with any sensitive topic, we can ruin our inquiry by rushing on without giving the patient time to consider the questions before answering. Silence will do its work if we allow it to.
   The current theory of intimate violence is that it is instrumental, i.e., used to control the victim. Nonetheless, asking about anger and the results of anger in the patient's life is a good way to uncover this particular family secret.

7. If you encounter syndromes (such as chronic pain or depression) that are often linked to a history of abuse, you can ask, "Some patients with your set of symptoms have been abused physically or sexually. To your knowledge, have you ever had those experiences? Has this ever happened to you?"

8. Once you have uncovered a history of violence in either the victim or the perpetrator, **remain empathic and nonjudgmental.** Ask what the patient has thought about the problem, what he or she has decided to do, and what sort of help you might give. Being nonjudgmental does not imply that you should not show your concern for the patient. Some doctors say they don't know what to say with victims of domestic violence. These have been suggested:

- "You did the right thing by telling me."
- "I'm glad you told me."
- "I'm sorry this happened to you."
- "This shouldn't be happening."
- "I'm concerned for your safety."
- "Are you safe right now?"
- "What do you think your options are?"
- "How can I help you?"
- "I have the phone numbers of some counselors. You can talk to them confidentially."

The National Domestic Violence Hotline is 800-799-7233. Call them for your local domestic violence resources.

Violence committed by intimates is a threat to health, and you should be familiar with available resources—safe house numbers, police numbers, and appropriate therapists. In some states the law requires that you report all violence-caused injuries. Be sure you know the law on reporting and have a protocol established.

PITFALLS TO AVOID

1. Forgetting violence—it's not a medical problem.

2. Addressing victimhood but forgetting the perpetrators.

3. Shaming and blaming victims and perpetrators of violence.

4. Uncovering the history of violence without knowing where help is available.

5. Arguing with your patient, insisting that he/she leave a dangerous relationship.

PEARL

Violence is a medical problem and a significant risk. Know about it and know the resources available to help.

SELECTED READINGS

Alpert EJ. Violence in intimate relationships and the practicing internist: new disease or new agenda? Ann Intern Med 1995;123: 774–778.

Bell CC. Community violence: causes, prevention and intervention. J Natl Med Assoc 1997;89:657–662.

Bullock KA, Schornstein SL. Improving medical care for victims of domestic violence. Hosp Physician 1998;23(9):42–57.

Herman JL. Trauma and recovery: the aftermath of violence—from domestic abuse to political terror. NY: Basic Books, 1992.

Hutson HR, Anglin D, Spears K. The perspectives of violent street gang injuries. Neurosurg Clin N Am 1995;6:621–628.

Lindsey M, McBride R, Platt CM. The third path: a workbook for ending violent behavior. Denver: Galantic Publishing, 1996.

Prothrow-Stith D. Deadly consequences: how violence is destroying our teenage population and a plan to begin solving the problem. NY: Harper, 1993.

Tavris C. Anger, the misunderstood emotion. NY: Touchstone Books, 1989.

Wilson-Brewer R, Spivak H. Violence prevention in schools and other community settings: the pediatrician as initiator, educator, collaborator and advocate. Pediatrics 1994;94:623–630.

Wright JL, Cheng TL. Successful approaches to community violence intervention and prevention. Pediatr Clin N Am 1998;45:459–467.

CHAPTER 28
Alcohol Use

PROBLEM

It's hard to determine when a patient's use of alcohol becomes abusive. One definition of alcohol abuse or addiction is continued use despite negative physical, psychologic, social, or economic consequences. It's not always easy to determine how much a patient drinks, much less whether the drinking is a problem.

> **Dr.:** So, Mr. B., do you drink?
>
> **Pt.:** Alcohol? You mean alcohol?
>
> **Dr.:** Yeah.
>
> **Pt.:** Oh, I don't hardly drink at all. Just a few beers.
>
> **Dr.:** Beers? How much?
>
> **Pt.:** Not that much. I'm no alcoholic or anything like that.
>
> **Dr.:** Well, how many in a week?
>
> **Pt.:** Oh, I don't keep track. Maybe two or three.
>
> **Dr.:** So two or three beers a week.
>
> **Pt.:** No, two or three a day. Usually I have a couple when I come home from work and maybe a couple later on or a few more on weekends, especially if I'm watching a football game.

So what's the standard? Is this patient a regular drinker, a problem drinker, a heavy drinker, an abuser of alcohol, or alcohol dependent? Can two or three drinks a day be part of a healthy life?

Alcohol treatment may be inpatient or outpatient, depending on the patient's level of function. Experts disagree about the best approach to treatment. But the physician's communication with the patient may have major effects on the patient's clinical outcome. Much of our recommended discourse regarding behavior change has already been covered in Chapters 16 and 25. This chapter will stress diagnosis.

PRINCIPLES

1. Alcohol and tobacco are the two most problematic legal drugs. They probably cause more injury, death, and illness than all the

illict drugs. A good method of discussing alcohol or tobacco use with your patient may serve equally well for talking about the use of illicit drugs such as heroin, cocaine, and amphetamines.

2. Our medical advice about alcohol use may be contradictory. Studies recommending alcohol use have been publicized in the popular press, but some authorities think that two drinks a day is "probable alcohol dependence," at least for women.

3. Many screening protocols and questionnaires are far too insensitive for reliable use in identifying problem drinkers. But they identify behaviors that will be familiar to patients, thus serve as good tools for introducing the subject of patients' alcohol use.

4. The physician's assessment of the patient's alcohol and drug use has to be done through conversation rather than with a bevy of case-defining questions.

5. Doctors may approach the alcoholic patient with a sense of hopelessness derived from their training experiences caring for patients with end-stage disease. However, physicians have good reasons to offer hope for recovery to patients whose disease is recognized early and who can work with approaches to behavior change.

6. Alcoholism is often viewed as a moral failing. The medical model views alcoholism as a treatable disorder and considers that the alcoholic patient, like most patients, is responsible for his/her choices about behavior in response to the disease. Many doctors are ambivalent about the medical model of alcoholism, however, and may hold both beliefs: that alcoholism is a treatable disease and that it is contracted by the morally weak. **As with all behavior disorders, alcoholism challenges our desire to determine responsibility for illness.**

PROCEDURES

1. **Inquire about alcohol use in your assessment of health risks,** although you may find that the patient's alcohol use is part of his or her social history as well. (He/she drinks in certain social situations with other drinking friends.) Inquire what and how much your patient drinks. Gently insist on as much precision as your patient can provide. For example, many patients don't consider use of beer or wine as "drinking," and may distinguish between expensive imported wine and domestic jug wine. In general, the more time it takes your patient to come up with an approximate amount of alcohol consumption, the more likely that alcohol is a significant problem to him/her.

2. Use the CAGE or a similar questionnaire to explore how the patient uses alcohol. Standardized questionnaires, research tools, and survey instruments can help guide the interview. Ask your patient:
    a) Are you or your friends and relatives concerned about your drinking? **Are you considering cutting down?**
    b) **Do you get angry** when I ask or others ask about your drinking? What other sorts of trouble is drinking causing?
    c) **Do you feel guilty** about drinking? Do you have bad feelings about problems that drinking caused or that it was associated with? Arrests? DUIs? Fights? Domestic violence? Bar fights? Illnesses related to alcohol?
    d) Do you take an "eye-opener," a drink first thing in the morning?
    e) When, what, how much do you drink? Teetotaler? Occasional drinker? More?

3. **Look for a positive answer to** item 2a, **"Are you considering cutting down?"** It signals the ambivalence of the contemplative stage of behavior change, and indicates that the patient may be ready to work with the doctor. After acknowledging the patient's ambivalence, we can ask him/her to make those two lists, the good things about drinking and the not-so-good things, and begin to plan how the patient might replace the benefits of drinking.

4. **Proceed to stage your patient in readiness to change his/her drinking behavior.** Question the patient about conviction and confidence, and match your intervention to this state. Does it help for the doctor to say something about the bad effects of drinking on the patient's health? Yes, surely, but using the tools of behavior change involves making the patient a partner in his recovery rather than imposing orders from above.

5. Remain optimistic. Don't let the patient's feelings of failure and hopelessness become your own.

PITFALLS TO AVOID

1. Failing to discuss alcohol use in our health assessment.

2. Trying to rescue or blame the patient.

3. Perpetuating the myth that an addict has no choices about his/her behavior

4. Allowing yourself to be co-opted by police and the legal system as an agent of punishment instead of healing.

5. Deferring to Alcoholics Anonymous instead of attempting to work with our patient ourselves. AA is helpful in maintaining sobriety, but doctors also have a role in treating addiction.

6. Failing to face our own addictive behavior, including alcoholism. Physicians are as susceptible to alcoholism and drug abuse as non-physicians.

PEARL

To understand your patient's alcohol or drug use, you must give the patient a conversation, not just a screening questionnaire.

SELECTED READINGS

Bradley KA. How much is too much? Advising patients about safe levels of alcohol consumption. Arch Intern Med 1993;153:2734–2740.

Bradley KA, Boyd-Wickizer J, Powell SH, Burman ML. Alcohol screening questionnaires in women. JAMA 1998;280:166–171.

Bradley KA, Bush KR, McDonell MB, Malone T, Fihn SD. Screening for problem drinking: comparison of CAGE and AUDIT. J Gen Intern Med 1988;13:379–388.

Conigliare J, Lofgren RP, Hanusa BH. Screening for problem drinking. Impact on physician behavior and patient drinking habits. J Gen Intern Med 1998;13:251–256.

Fleming MF, Barry KL, Manwell LB, Johnson K, London R. Brief physician advice for problem alcohol drinkers. JAMA 1987;277:1039–1045.

Johnson B, Clark W. Alcoholism: a challenging physician–patient encounter. J Gen Intern Med 1989;4:445–452.

Steinweg D. Alcoholism: the keys to the cage. Am J Med 1993;94:520–523.

Wallace P, Cutler S, Haines A. Randomized controlled trial of general practitioner intervention in patients with excessive alcohol consumption. BMJ 1988;297:663–668.

Zweben JE, Clark HW. Unrecognized substance misuse: clinical hazards and legal vulnerabilities. Int J Addict 1990–1991;25:1431–1451.

CHAPTER 29

Sex

PROBLEM

Sexuality provides humankind with great pleasure and great pain. Part of the pain arises from our general inability to deal with sexual matters in the context of health. As physicians, we have to inquire about our patients' sexual behaviors. Since sexual behaviors tend to be kept private, both we and our patients may be reticent about broaching the subject.

PRINCIPLES

1. Sexual activity is a normal part of health-related behavior.

2. Physicians can be helpful to their patients in addressing sexual dysfunction and risk.

3. Patients are hesitant to broach the subject, but doctors must.

4. Our inquiry should include risks of sexually transmitted disease and sexual dysfunction.

5. In dealing with patients' sex-related health issues, we will sometimes have difficult judgments to make about confidentiality. If we fail to enter data in the record, we may forget important information. If we do enter it, the information becomes accessible to others. We also have problems with sexually transmittable disease (STD) contact notification. If we are caring for both partners in a relationship and one develops a sexually transmittable disease, we encounter ethical and legal problems relating to disclosure.

PROCEDURES

1. **Preface discussion of sensitive topics with an explanation about your need to explore into private areas:** "These are questions I always ask my patients. Because of the hazard of sexually transmitted diseases these days, doctors have to discuss more than we used to in areas many patients usually keep private. I am going to ask you some questions about sexuality." Two simple questions may be adequate to gather the data you need: "Are you sexually active?" and "Are you having any sexual difficulties or problems at this time?"

2. **Ask your patient about sexual partners.** Be prepared for the usual possibilities, including heterosexuality, homosexuality, bisexuality, and sex aids. **Listen without judgment.**

3. **Ask about the kind of protection against disease or injury your patient uses.**

4. **Be matter of fact:**

> **Dr.:** (to herself) This is part of my usual database. I always ask these questions.
>
> **Dr.:** (to her patient) Part of the health exam includes information about sexual behavior and risks. May I ask you a couple of questions?
>
> **Pt.:** I guess so.
>
> **Dr.:** Are you sexually active?
>
> **Pt.:** Not much lately.
>
> **Dr.:** Are you content with your sex life, or are there any problems?

Of course, being matter-of-fact about this inquiry does not mean you should trample over your patient's feelings. In fact the patient's feelings of discomfort should be addressed just as you address other distresses, with empathy. You will have to introduce the issue of sexual hazards: "Some kinds of sexual behavior carry more risks than others, so I will ask you about those."

5. Sexual function includes desire, erection, and ejaculation in men; and desire, lubrication, sensation, and climax in women. **We can ask about function and satisfaction.** Sexual problems cited by patients include: concern about frequency of intercourse, lack of sexual desire, marital or relationship problems, sexual problems related to illness, lack of orgasm, concern about sexual orientation, painful intercourse, lack of knowledge about sexual function or hazards, premature ejaculations, traumatic past sexual experiences, erectile dysfunction, contraceptive needs, concerns about masturbation, and extramarital relationships.

6. **Be aware of your own biases** about normal sexual practices, and try not to curtail discussion or impose judgement when you become uncomfortable.

167

Dr.: (to himself): I'd never want to do what this guy does. How does he stand it? Better take this slowly and remember it's his life.

Dr.: (to patient): Whips, eh?

7. **Listen for the patient's initiation of talk about sexuality and follow up on it.**

Pt.: I went through a tiny promiscuous phase.

Dr.: I see. Tell me more about that.

Much better than fleeing the issue, as Epstein quotes:

Dr.: Just a tiny phase, eh? OK, what other problems do you have?

Be alert to behaviors that block communication: premature closure, forgetting or ignoring patient concerns, failing to pursue discussion of sexuality and sexually transmitted diseases, and lack of response to patient distress signals. Most of our avoidance probably stems from our own discomfort with the topic, so the best corrective is to identify and suppress our own discomforts. Remaining sensitive to these interviewing behaviors may help too.

8. **Persevere.** Don't stop your inquiry until you have adequate answers.

Dr.: Any concerns or questions about sexuality?

Pt.: Just lack of, no. (laughter)

Dr.: Oh, lack thereof. (laughs) OK.

We often ask questions, fail to get an answer, and go on as if we had been satisfied in our inquiry. Ask again until you do get an answer. If you move on to another area before you understand the answers to your questions, you will miss important data:

Dr.: Have you ever had any sexually transmitted diseases?

Pt.: Not exactly, no. At least not for sure.

Dr.: OK. On to the next question on my list. How about seat belts? Use them in the car?

This doctor has to find out what "not exactly" and "not for sure" mean. A number of patients don't know what sexually transmitted diseases are, so a short list is helpful. "Have you ever had any sexually transmitted diseases like herpes? Gonorrhea?" pausing after each name to elicit an answer.

PITFALLS TO AVOID

1. Avoiding the topic, especially if the patient is older than you or is married.
   (60-year-olds don't have sex, do they? Married people don't have extramarital sex, do they?)

2. Asking half-hearted questions; failing to follow up ambiguous answers.

3. Disregarding your own discomfort and that of your patient.

4. Expressing disgust, fascination, or disbelief at your patient's account of sexual behavior.

PEARL

Patient behavior includes sexual behavior. Ask.

SELECTED READINGS

Bachmann GA, Leiblum SR, Grill J. Brief sexual inquiry in gynecologic practice. Obstet Gynecol 1989;73:425–427.
Bullard DG, Caplan HW. Sexual problems. In: Feldman MD, Christensen JF, eds. Behavioral medicine in primary care. Stamford, CT: Appleton and Lange, 1997:247–264.
Ende J, Rockwell S, Glasgow M. The sexual history in general medical practice. Arch Intern Med 1984;144:558–561.
Epstein RM et al. Awkward moments in patient–physician communication about HIV risk. Ann Intern Med 1998;128:435–442.
Simkin RJ. Not all your patients are straight. JAMC 1998;159: 370–374.

White JC, Levinson W. Lesbian health care: what a primary care physician needs to know. West J Med 1995;162:463–466.

Williams S. The sexual history. In: Lipkin M, Putnam SM, Lazare A, eds. The medical interview. clinical care, education and research. NY: Springer-Verlag, 1995:235–250.

Part VI
Frequent Problems

CHAPTER 30
The List-Maker

PROBLEM

All over the world, doctors quail when patients bring lists. Why? Don't we all write lists for ourselves? We probably find the list frustrating because we lack control over the patient's report of its contents, which are often disorganized and unprioritized.

PRINCIPLES

1. The dreaded list is a gift in disguise, a rough draft of the patient's agenda that we encourage you to find. You can convert the unhelpful list into a helpful one by working with the patient to group related problems and identify the most important ones.

2. When you realize that you have a list-making patient, you can help him/her help you. Suggest a format for the list, or recommend ways the patient can record health data. This may turn up important information for the next history.

PROCEDURES

1. Be aware of any immediate negative response you might have to a list and get beyond it. **Reframe "The List" as an aid to your work.**

2. **Explain what you need from your patient.**

> **Dr.:** A really useful list requires time to prepare. Do make a list, by all means, but please give it some thought. Start with a list that includes everything you want to talk to me about, then star the two most important items. Then please make another copy so when you come in, we each can have one to look at.

Does that work? Sure. When one of the authors goes to see his doctor he brings just that sort of a list. And he tries to introduce the list gently to his doctor:

> **Pt.:** John, I don't want to scare you, but ....
>
> **Dr.:** Scare me? What do you mean?   *continued*

> **Pt.:** Well, I brought a list.
>
> **Dr.:** A list?
>
> **Pt.:** Yes, but I think I've got it well-organized, and I don't really expect that we'll be able to deal with more than the first two topics. And I brought two copies. Here's yours.

3. Put the list in the chart so the patient feels heard, and so you can refer back to it at the next visit in case you didn't cover all the topics.

PITFALLS TO AVOID

1. Disregarding your patient's list and his/her list-making efforts.

2. Struggling with the patient for control of the interview agenda.

3. Failing to educate your patient about how he/she can best help you to help him/her.

PEARL

A good list is a blessing.

SELECTED READINGS

Beckman HB, Frankel RM. The effect of physician behavior on the collection of data. Ann Intern Med 1984;101:692–696.

Joos SK, Hickam DH, Gordon GH, Baker LH. Effects of a physician communication intervention on patient care outcomes. J Gen Intern Med 1996;11:147–155.

Keller VF, Carroll JG. A new model for physician–patient communication. Patient Educ Couns 1994;23:131–140.

Lazare A, Eisenthal S, Wasserman L. The customer approach to patient-hood: attending to patient requests in a walk-in clinic. Arch Gen Psychiatry 1975;32:553–558.

Platt F. The dreaded list. Patient Care 1997;31(4):122–125

Starfield B, Wray C, Hess K, Gross R, Birk PS, D-Lugoff BC. The influence of patient–practitioner agreement on outcome of care. Am J Public Health 1981;71:127–31.

White J, Levinson W, Roter D. Oh, by the way: the closing moments of the medical visit. J Gen Intern Med 1994;9:24–8.

CHAPTER 31

The Patient's Companion

PROBLEM

When the patient is accompanied by a friend or relative, we're often unclear about that companion's function in the interview. We question whom we should listen to, and whether we should turn the companion out of the interview room. However, we realize that asking a companion to go might not work if he/she refused to leave.

> **Dr.:** Hi, Mr. and Mrs. B. I'm Dr. X. I understand Mr. B. is here today with some breathing trouble.
>
> **Wife:** That's right, doctor. He just huffs and puffs. Sometimes I really get worried. He makes all those sounds.
>
> **Dr.:** What does it feel like to you, Mr. B.?
>
> **Pt.:** Well, I'm OK, I think.
>
> **Wife:** Horace, how can you say that when you cough and sputter so? (to doctor:) He never tells the doctors anything. That's why I have to come with him.
>
> **Dr.:** It would help me to hear from Mr. B., though. Mrs. B., perhaps you could wait until we are done and then fill in the blanks.
>
> **Wife:** OK, doctor.
>
> **Dr.:** So tell me what else is troubling you.
>
> **Pt.:** Nothing much.
>
> **Wife:** His legs swell up.

This sort of trialogue bothers doctors. What sort of strategy would work best?

PRINCIPLES

1. We still should make a serious **effort to address the patient first, and only involve the companion after asking permission of the patient.** We don't want to break up a tight unit, but we must see and talk with the patient to uncover diagnoses.

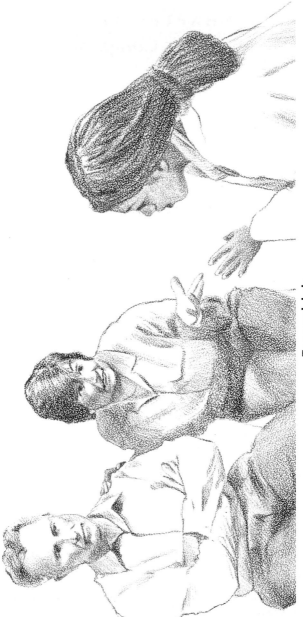

Too much help

2. Despite our desires to first deal with the patient alone, we often find ourselves stuck with both members of the team. Although the companion who wants a role in the medical interview challenges the physician's control, he/she may be a blessing in disguise. The patient may be confused, delirious, or forgetful. **This helper may be the only source of medical data available.** Or, true to gender stereotypes, the male in the family may be the strong silent type who relies on his wife to express emotion and convey information about needs.

3. It might help to imagine that the second person is the caretaker who is trying to introduce his/her patient to you, not to dominate the interaction. When the spouse is the patient's caretaker, the doctor should respect that role and consider himself/herself a consultant to that primary caretaker. Hear the caretaker's story first.

4. When an identified patient is accompanied by an intimate, you may have two patients in the room. In this case, one is suffering from cough and dyspnea, the other from fears and worries, or perhaps with anger at the identified patient. If so, **you may have to deal with the more voluble patient first.**

5. Finally you should consider the possibility that the second person is present to prevent the truth from being uttered. Spousal abusers sometimes accompany their mate to the doctor to prevent the story of abuse from being told and being heard.

PROCEDURES

1. Start with your usual procedure, listening first to the identified patient.

> **Dr.:** Mrs. and Mr. B., what usually works best for me is to hear from the patient first and then ask his companion to fill in the blanks. Would that work here?
>
> **Wife:** I doubt it, doctor. He never tells doctors anything, and now he's so short of breath that he answers everything with just a word or two. But I've been caring for him for 48 years and I can tell you what's going on.
>
> **Dr.:** That sounds important for me to hear. Can I first ask him to tell me his symptoms though? He's the only one who really can say just how he feels.

2. If that doesn't work, you can try a three-step process, explaining the entire plan to both participants. The first step is to ask the companion to step out, saying that you will join him/her later. Next, still with the patient, you should ask if the patient or his/her companion left anything unsaid so far and then ask the patient for permission to share information with the companion. Once you move out of the room to talk with the companion, you have to inquire about the companion's concerns, questions, and ideas. That is, you really turn your attention to the companion. Finally you bring the two back together and share fears and ideas. You can work towards a discussion of problems and disagreements.

> **Dr.:** Mrs. B., what I'd like to do is have you step out and wait a bit in the waiting room. I'll be back with you later. Then, Mr. B., I'd like to examine you. Afterwards I will come get your wife and we can all talk together. OK?

That might work. You plan to test your patient's ability to give data and to form a rapport with you. You will ask him what he wants you to say to his wife and if there is anything he does not want you to say. Then you can bring her back in and continue the discussion.

3. Another approach is to assume you have two patients and ask the second patient how she is doing. Note that you are not asking her to tell her husband's story, but her own.

> **Dr.:** Mrs. B., before we talk more about your husband, I want to ask you a little about how this has been going for you. You said you two have been together for 50 years.
>
> **Wife:** Almost. Almost 50 years. And he's always been so healthy until these last three years.
>
> **Dr.:** So you've been caring for him.
>
> **Wife:** I do. I'm the one who takes care at home.
>
> **Dr.:** And you've been worrying about him?
>
> **Wife:** I worry so much, doctor. My brother has lung cancer and we don't know how long he'll last. Now I worry about both of them. John here is all I've got. We need each other.

continued

> **Dr.:** I see. You're worried that he might get so sick that he'd die but because John doesn't complain much, we'd miss it.
>
> **Wife:** That's it, Doctor.

4. Once you've heard a little about the companion, ask him or her to tell you the most important problems of your identified patient before you try to interview him/her again. Then perhaps you can defer talking with the identified patient until it is physical exam time, a good time to invite the spouse to leave the room with a promise that you will have him/her in again when you are finished. Few companions will hang around at rectal-exam time.

PITFALLS TO AVOID

1. Trying to crash through the interview despite the companion's interruptions.

2. Getting angry at the interfering party.

3. Missing the important information the caretaker can contribute.

4. Failing to see you have two patients, not one.

PEARL

An interfering companion can be a second patient clamoring for your attention and/or a source of information about the identified patient. Maybe both!

SELECTED READINGS

Adelman RD, Greene MG, Charon R. The physician–elderly patient–companion triad in the medical encounter: the development of a conceptual framework and research agenda. Gerontologist 1987: 27:729–734.

Botelho RJ, Lue BH, Fiscella K. Family involvement in routine health care: a survey of patients' behaviors and preferences. J Fam Pract 1996;42:572–576.

Brown JB, Brett P, Steward M, Marshall JN. Roles and influence of people who accompany patients on visits to the doctor. Can Fam Physician 1998;44:1644–1650.

Campbell TL, McDaniel SH. Conducting Family Interviews. In: Lipkin M, Putnam SM, Lazare A, eds. The medical interview: clinical care, education and research. NY: Springer-Verlag, 1995;173–189.

Finger AL. Enlisting a patient's adult children as allies. Med Economics 1997;74(3):173–189.

Greene MG, Majerovitz SD, Adelman RD, Rizzo C. The effects of the presence of a third person on the physician–older patient medical interview. J Am Geriatr Soc 1994;42:413–419.

Hahn S, Feiner JS, Belling EH. The doctor–patient–family relationship: a compensatory alliance. Ann Intern Med 1988;109:884–889.

Hang MR. Elderly patients, caregivers and physicians: theory and research on healthcare triads. J Health Soc Behav 1994;35:1–12.

Herlman SC, Witztum E. Patients, chaperons and healers: enlarging the therapeutic encounter. Soc Sci Med 1994;39:133–143.

Platt FW. Lots of help. In: Conversation failure: case studies in doctor–patient communication. Tacoma: Life Sciences Press, 1992: 20–23.

CHAPTER 32

Confusion: Communicating With the Cognitively Impaired Patient

PROBLEM

Many of our patients are globally confused, suffering from cognitive dysfunction with defects of orientation, attention, thinking, and memory. We find many such patients in hospital work. We encounter three major syndromes:

a) Delirium, a disorder of thinking, orientation, and memory that begins acutely and may vary from hour to hour. We may find our patient in a lucid interval and miss the diagnosis.

b) Dementia, a chronic progressive condition that may leave social skills intact. Such a patient may be quite attentive and may retain remote memory, but be quite confused about current happenings in his life.

c) Strokes, trauma, and congenital defects that produce chronic and stable brain defects.

In all these situations, as we try to interview our patient, the interview may simply replicate that confusion. Our first challenge is to realize that the patient is too mixed up to give a straight story.

PRINCIPLES

1. We underestimate the degree of cognitive impairment that many patients have. Many medical conditions can produce some degree of cognitive impairment.

2. When things aren't going well in the interview, think about the possibility of cognitive impairment. You may find the patient's story confusing, incomplete, or contradictory, leading you to label him/her a "poor historian."

Or you may find it hard to develop your usual degree of rapport with the patient. Confused patients can be hostile and uncooperative, agitated and anxious, or withdrawn and avoidant. Some may use politeness or humor to hide their confusion.

3. If you suspect that the patient is confused, guide the interview into an assessment for confusion. Discovering confusion will keep you from sinking into a morass of noninformation, simply demonstrating that confusion again and again and expecting a degree of precision and rapport that the patient cannot provide.

4. Become familiar with a mental status examination for evaluation of confusion.

PROCEDURES

1. If you are uncomfortable because of data imprecision or lack of a working relationship with your patient, stop and consider the possibility of cognitive impairment.

2. Begin by checking for precision in the history: How long ago was that? What year was that? How old were you then? Was that before or after your surgery? You can check on the facts from the chart to compare with what your patient tells you.

3. Prepare the patient for the mental status exam. Asking about memory usually is least traumatic:

> **Dr.:** Mr. A., lots of people with medical problems like yours have trouble with their memory. How has your memory been doing?
>
> **Pt.:** Not so hot, Doctor. Sometimes I forget names.
>
> **Dr.:** Well, that's understandable. Let me ask you some questions to understand just how well your memory works.
>
> **Pt.:** OK.

4. The Mini-Mental Status Exam described by Folstein and colleagues is quite popular and well standardized (Folstein, 1975). Another Organic Mental Status Exam that we find useful was described by Jacobs et al. (Jacobs, 1977). These tests look at attention, perception, orientation, both short- and long-term memory, calculation, and judgment, and give you a quantitative estimate of the patient's function.

5. Once you've identified cognitive dysfunction, try to adjust your team's efforts to provide care. Patients often need frequent orientation, assistance and predictable routines. They will respond more to your tone of voice and body language than your reasoning and logic.

    With all these patients respect is important and empathy for their struggle and their discomfort will help greatly.

PITFALLS TO AVOID

1. Missing confusion. Patients become adept at covering it up, usually with jesting, sometimes with anger.

> **Dr.:** Are you having any trouble with your memory? Do you remember who I am?
>
> **Pt.:** Of course I do. You're the same guy you used to be.

2. Continuing to try to get data from a patient who is unable to convey a sensible story.

3. Failing to consider the diagnostic alternatives: dementia, psychosis, delirium, aphasia, and developmental disability.

PEARL

Remember that the patient's confusion may be part of the story.

SELECTED READINGS

Folstein MF, Folstein SF, McHugh PR. Mini-Mental state examination. J Psychiatr Res 1975;12:189–198.

Inouye SK. The dilemma of delerium: clinical and research controversies regarding diagnosis and evaluation of delerium in hospitalized elderly medical patients. Am J Med 1994;97:278–288.

Jacobs JW, Bernhard MR, Delgado A, Strain JJ. Screening for organic mental syndromes in the medically ill. Ann Intern Med 1977;86: 40–46.

Lipowski ZJ. Update on delirium. Psychiatr Clin North Am 1992;15: 335–346.

McEvoy JP. Organic brain syndromes. Ann Intern Med 1981;95: 212–220.

CHAPTER 33
The New HMO Patient

PROBLEM

While HMOs cast primary care physicians in the role of gatekeeper, many of their patients view them as rubber stamps for approving referrals. At the same time, subspecialists complain that patients they have cared for over many years now have to be screened by a primary physician who hardly knows them, may be unfamiliar with their medical issues, and may lack the expertise to decide when a referral is needed.

The most common difficulties physicians cite with HMO medicine are a) requests for automatic referrals to subspecialists, b) the angry patient who has had to leave a trusted doctor because of insurance changes, and c) HMO clerks' interference in referrals, prescribing, and tasks of care.

PRINCIPLES

1. Your first task—as always—is to remain calm. The patient did not create the problem he's bringing to you, and his request reflects ignorance of what doctors do rather than disrespect of your medical expertise.

2. Your task is always to **engage the patient**, using procedures that connect the two of you professionally and also as two human beings.

3. The very concept of a primary care physician may be foreign to your patient. You may have to explain your function, not just what you don't or won't do, but what you can and will do for the patient.

4. Remember that although you are a commodity to HMOs, to the suffering patient who needs your skills at examination and diagnosis, you are a doctor. A careful history and physical examination can calm and satisfy both parties.

5. The patient may find the demands of managed care as new and as problematic as you do. He or she may also be feeling anger, sadness, or embarrassment. Finding out how the patient feels and letting him/her know that you understand that feeling are part of the treatment of a referral-seeker.

PROCEDURES

1. Acknowledge to yourself how you are feeling and control your responses to those feelings. An interior dialogue may help.

2. **Employ engagement techniques.** Your goal is to develop an implicit contract in which you both agree on roles, rules of discourse, and agendas.
    a) **Inquire about and attend to the person of the patient.**

Dr.: Mr. B., we haven't worked together before, and before we talk about referrals for your knee and your stomach, I need to get to know you a little. Could you tell me about yourself as a person?

Pt.: Huh? Well, what do you want to know?

Dr.: Oh, how you spend your time, what other people are in your life, what's important to you and to your health.

Pt.: Well, I'm married. We have two daughters in high school. I work as an actuary—that's a sort of glorified accountant. I'm from Baltimore, but I've been out here for almost 20 years now.

(pause)

Dr.: Anything else?

Pt.: Not much. I am pretty athletic still, like to ski and play tennis. And I read a lot, mostly history books.

(pause)

Dr.: So married, two daughters, actuary, athletic, and a reader of history!

Pt.: That's it, Doc. That's me.

Dr.: OK, then how about telling me about your health?

Note how effortlessly this interview segues into the usual medical interview format. That's what we mean by suggesting that you remember to do doctoring and note that doctoring itself is very comforting to patients.

b) **Explore the patient's agenda.**

> **Dr.:** So you're here for referrals to your orthopedist and your gastroenterologist. Tell me what other issues or problems or concerns you have today.

c) **Discuss your agenda and the differences between the two.**

> **Dr.:** Mr. B. Sounds like you're primarily here for referrals to those other doctors and that you are doing pretty well but you've been gaining some weight and are concerned about it, and you've noted that you don't ever seem to get enough sleep anymore. Is that about it?
>
> **Pt.:** That's it, doctor. In a nutshell.
>
> **Dr.:** OK, as your new primary care doctor I need to explain what my role is and then I ought to do a quick general examination so I know what you look like when you're feeling well, then I ought to pay attention to the weight issue and the sleepiness issue.
>
> **Pt.:** Well I hadn't planned all that but it sounds OK to me.

d) **Then do a careful history and physical examination.**

3. **Where differences of role expectations exist, articulate those differences and discuss them.**

> **Dr.:** I see. Well, sounds like we have somewhat different views of my role. If I understand you correctly, you think I should write out referrals to your bone and stomach doctors. On the other hand, I think my job is to come to know you, review your medical history, and do a careful physical examination. Then, depending on what we find and what you and I decide to do, consider what comes next, possibly some referrals to subspecialists. So we have different ideas of what I need to do for you first.

Once you've done all this, your patient's initial plan may have changed to resemble yours. But you need to check.

> **Dr.:** There is one more thing. I remember that you came seeking referrals to several other doctors and now, after my examination, I've suggested that you're doing fine and don't need to see them. How do you feel about that?

Such a request will allow the patient to tell you that he's angry, still worried, or content. If he's still distressed, you may need to hear more about that and let the patient know that you hear him, that you can understand, that his distress makes sense to you, and that you may be willing to negotiate on the matter. I suspect this patient will be quite content.

4. Use empathic communication for troubled patient feelings.

> **Dr.:** Hello Mr. Cinch., I'm Dr. X. I'm glad to meet you.
>
> **Pt.:** Hello, Doctor. I'm here because my company changed insurance. I don't know why I had to leave Dr. Y. He was really good. He was my doctor for five years. I hate having to switch.
>
> **Dr.:** So your company changed programs and your doctor wasn't on the new one and you got me instead. It must be a drag to have to leave a doctor you liked and trusted just because of an insurance change.
>
> **Pt.:** It is, doctor. I don't have anything against you.
>
> **Dr.:** Of course you don't. But still, you don't know me, don't yet know if you can trust me as you did Dr. Y. That's hard for you.
>
> **Pt.:** Yeah. But anyway, since I'm here, I guess you'll do. At least you understand.
>
> **Pt.:** Thanks.

Of all the words a patient can say, this minimal thank-you, this "at least you understand," sounds best to us. If we hear it we know we have done our job, and the process of building an alliance with Mr. C. has begun.

What do you think of this dialogue? What happened? First of all, the doctor didn't react with anger or hurt feelings to the patient's complaint about having him as a new doctor. Then the doctor strove to understand the patient's feeling that accompanied his complaint. A little bit of understanding, well communicated, can go a long way.

PITFALLS TO AVOID

1. Teaming up with your patient to bash the HMO.

2. Ignoring your own emotions during the encounter.

3. Failing to control your imagination. Worrying most about what you imagine to be about to happen, e.g., that dealing with the problem will take a long time.

PEARL

Keep your eye on the prize: the tasks of doctoring.

SELECTED READINGS

Emanuel EJ, Dubler NN. Preserving the physician–patient relationship in the era of managed care. JAMA 1995;273(4):323–329.

Gordon GH, Baker L, Levinson W. Physician–patient communication in managed care. West J Med 1995;163:43–47.

Mechanic D, Schlesinger M. The impact of managed care on patients' trust in medical care and their physicians. JAMA 1996;275: 1693–1697.

Platt F. I'm here for a referral. *Patient Care* 1997;31(1):143–144.

Schroeder JL, Clark JT, Webster JR. Prepaid entitlements: a new challenge for physician–patient relationships. JAMA 1985;254(21): 3080–3082.

CHAPTER 34
The Patient Bearing Literature

PROBLEM

Patients have always brought newspaper and magazine clippings, testimonials, and advertisements to their doctors. In recent decades, medical information available to patients has increased significantly in amount and sophistication. Organizations providing patient information, support, and advocacy are expanding, and print and broadcast media regularly feature medical news. At least one-third of U.S. homes are equipped with personal computers, and seeking medical information is a common reason to log on to the internet. Patients with internet access can draw on a variety of health-related web sites, journal searches, bulletin boards, chat rooms, and informal advisors.

There are many positive aspects to a patient bringing medical news into the office. The news can reinforce knowledge and skills relevant to self-care and promote attitudes of personal responsibility for health. Sometimes the source of the news becomes a social support system for the patient. At times popular media may reach patients before professional media reaches doctors, such that patients may be better informed than their doctors about some issues.

There are also negative aspects. The patient may bring in a large quantity of information that needs to be organized and put into perspective. Information on the internet is poorly regulated, and information about diagnoses, tests, or treatments may be unproven or dangerous. Some promising procedures turn out to be available only locally to patients who are part of a clinical trial. Our patients seldom can distinguish good information from unsupported advertising of bogus cures. But they all need you to credit their industry and their information.

> **Pt.:** (Flourishing something about The Yeast Beast) Doctor, have you read this book? It describes me to a "T."

> **Pt.:** Did you see that program last night? The one where they said there was something new for something like what I've got?

> **Pt.:** I brought some material from the internet. I found 1840 references to fibromyositis last night.

PRINCIPLES

1. Regardless of the quantity and quality of information that patients bring to the visit, premature dismissal or rejection of the information or process can trigger shame or anger, and undermine your efforts to help chronically ill patients self-manage their diseases more effectively. Credit the patient, not necessarily the material.

2. Explain and adhere to your usual procedures. That's the platform you're going to stand on. Obtain a careful and symptomatic history, do a careful physical examination, insist on diagnosis before therapy. Once you have your own data about the patient, you will have a much better grasp on the best next route to follow and your patient will be considerably reassured by your efforts to carefully understand him and his problems.

3. Whether the patient's information is valid or not, and regardless of education, profession, and other technical sophistication, your patient may lack enough basic biology knowledge—anatomy, physiology, pathology—to adequately use that information. You will have to educate him.

4. Our goal is to establish a partnership with our patient in the quest for further information and better education.

5. Consider becoming familiar with recurrent themes or requests.

> **Dr.:** Mr. X., I'm glad you brought me this book on "The Yeast Beast." A few years ago there was a study done to test how well the treatment described in this book would work. The patients who got the treatment did no better than those who didn't, even though they had the symptoms this book describes. We try to stay current on this topic because other patients ask about it too.

6. Once you review the material, if you decide it is not related to your work with the patient, be able to explain how it differs from your approach.

> **Dr.:** Mrs. P., this article is talking about an old approach to healing that I don't practice. I practice what is called evidence-based medicine or scientific medicine. It's only a couple of hundred of years old, pretty new compared to the more traditional faith-based approaches such as this article talks about. If you decide to work with a practitioner of this approach, please do let me know so I will know what you are doing, but what I have to offer is different.

PROCEDURES

1. Acknowledge and appreciate the act of bringing information in
    and asking about it. The patient is trying to become a more in-
    formed, active participant.

> **Dr.:** I can see that you spent quite a bit of time on this. I really
> appreciate your working to understand and sort out these trou-
> bles you've been having. How did you experience the search
> on the internet? I've found it hard sometimes myself to distin-
> guish important material from other stuff.

2. Acknowledge the content of the information. Thank the patient
    for bringing it to your attention. If the information looks trouble-
    some or complicated, tell the patient you'd like some time to re-
    view it before discussing it with him, and don't let it interfere
    with your time with the patient. You're going to have to look at
    the literature. Don't forget that your patient may actually have
    found something that you don't know!

> **Pt.:** I hear there is a new drug for diabetes that might help me
> lose weight.
>
> **Dr.:** Don't be ridiculous!

    This doctor was later surprised to discover that such a drug was
indeed just available, metformin hydrochloride (Glucophage). He
had a lot of apologizing to do.

3. Be sure to ask the patient what he learned from the information,
    and how he thinks it might apply to his care. Ask what he would
    like you to pay particular attention to as you look through the
    material. This step is key to helping the patient become a
    thoughtful and discriminating observer of his condition, as well
    as of relevant information. Document your patients information
    in the chart much as you would his ideas of the correct diagnosis
    or therapy.

4. Introduce your explanations by asking your patient for his under-
    standing of the anatomy and physiology involved. Then begin
    where he needs help.

5. If you have negative comments about the information, hold them
    until you've done your own work. Take a history, examine the

patient, formulate some hypotheses, and discuss them with the patient. Only then might it be time to discuss the troublesome information.

PITFALLS TO AVOID

1. Denigrating the patient's information and his very efforts to self-educate.

> **Dr.:** This stuff isn't worth the paper it's printed on.
>
> **Pt.:** But I spent a lot of time on the net last night, and there is a lot of information there.
>
> **Dr.:** Well you really wasted your time. You would have done better watching the football game.

2. Entering into a contest of authority.

3. Forgetting to do your own careful diagnostic medical work, rushing to address your patient's new source of information before you take a history or do an examination.

PEARL

Credit the patient whether you do or don't credit his information.

SELECTED READINGS

Culver JD, Gerr F, Frumkin H. Medical information on the internet: study of an electronic bulletin board. J Gen Intern Med 1997;12: 466–470.

Mandl KD, Kohane IS, Brandt AM. Electronic patient–physician communication: problems and promise. Ann Intern Med 1998;129: 495–500.

McClung HJ, Murray RD, Hilinger LA. The internet as a source for current patient information. Pediatrics 1998;101:E2

CHAPTER 35
Distant Medicine

PROBLEM

We are often asked to perform examinations and provide therapy at a distance. We may even seek such contacts. But when we don't have other real physical face-to-face contacts with the patient, all medicine at a distance remains dangerous.

> **Pt.:** (by phone) Doctor, I have this new rash and I was hoping you could call something in for it.
>
> **Dr.:** What does it look like?
>
> **Pt.:** Just a rash, doctor. It's just a rash. I think I had something like it once before.
>
> **Dr.:** Well, hold it up to the phone so I can get a look at it.

About 20% of primary care physicians' contacts with patients are made by phone. The calls typically last only a few minutes. During that time the doctor has to decide how serious the problem is, how urgently the patient has to be seen, and whether or not treatment should start before the patient is seen. These decisions involve a balance of context (distance from the doctor, the patient's ability to describe and monitor signs and symptoms, the degree of anxiety and social support) and content. The doctor must consider the potential seriousness of the symptoms in this patient and whether or not he can rapidly develop a hypothesis based on these limited data.

Nowadays, electronic mail is taking over for phone calls. And phone calls often turn out to be a matter of trading messages by phone mail. Some physicians and patients already communicate by e-mail. Such communication may serve well for general or patient-specific information, for reminders for appointments and screening procedures, for gathering routine data, and for checking back on a patient's status. But e-mail seldom can be depended on for exchange of urgent or complicated information that may not be noted in a timely way and may easily be misunderstood by either party.

PRINCIPLES

1. Telephone medicine may be an inevitable part of your practice, but it is fraught with uncertainty. Your diagnoses will be more intuitive and triagelike, and will always suffer from the absence of direct observations and examination data. Beware.

2. Electronic mail does provide time for reflection. While medicine practiced over e-mail means working deprived of your senses, the thoughtfulness of the obligatory pauses may be a help.

3. Phone follow-up can be a great help. The use of phone and e-mail can improve the relationship between doctor and patient. Routine calls in one study reduced the need for scheduled visits without increasing the rate of unscheduled visits or causing any increase in morbidity.

> **Dr.:** (by phone) Hi Charley, how is that cough doing?
>
> **Pt.:** Much better, doctor. With the antibiotic you prescribed day before yesterday it's practically gone.
>
> **Dr.:** Great! That's just what I hoped to hear.
>
> **Pt.:** Thanks for calling, doctor. I appreciate it.
>
> **Dr.:** You're welcome. I'll see you at that next appointment. Bye.

PROCEDURES

1. Your phone triage may include questions such as how sick the patient feels or looks, what the patient's temperature is, and discussion of what signs should worry the patient or the patient's parent.

2. Explain your needs carefully to your patient.

> **Dr.:** Mr. A., I appreciate that you've got this new rash and that you need some help for it, but I can't do much without a look at it. I think you and your rash have to come in so I can see it.

3. You can define your boundaries so as to remain within the confines of good and safe medical care.

> **Dr.:** I always insist on examining a patient who has a cough and sore throat like yours before prescribing an antibiotic or any other medicines. That's the way I work.

4. If you do prescribe treatment by phone, be careful to precisely arrange follow-up visits and to document your conversations in the chart the next day.

PITFALLS TO AVOID

1. Accepting the easy way out. Freely giving medical advice and prescriptions without the one-on-one contact that assures good care.

2. Assuming that modern technology like e-mail can replace older technology like chest auscultation.

PEARL

Phones and e-mail are best used to enhance but not replace a face-to-face encounter.

SELECTED READINGS

Balas EA, Jaffrey F, Kuperman GJ, Boren SA, Brown GD, Pinciroli F, Mitchell JA. Electronic communication with patients. Evaluation of distance medicine technology. JAMA 1997;278:152–159.

Borowitz SM, Wyatt JC. The origin, content, and workload of E-mail consultations. JAMA 1998;280:1321–1324.

Curtis P. The practice of medicine on the telephone. J Gen Intern Med 1988;3:294–296.

Mandl KD, Cohane IF, Brandt AM. Electronic patient–physician communication: problems and promise. Ann Intern Med 1998;129:495–500.

Pal B. Following up outpatients by telephone: a pilot study. Brit Med J: 1998;316:1647.

Peters RM. After-hours telephone calls to general and subspecialty internists: an observational study. J Gen Intern Med 1994;10:554–557.

Robinson TN, Patrick K, Eng TR, Gustafson D. An evidence-based approach to interactive health communication: a challenge to medicine in the information age. JAMA 98;280:1264–1269.

Spielberg AR. On call and online: sociohistorical, legal, and ethical implications of E-mail for the patient–physician relationship. JAMA 1998;280:1353–1359.

Wasson J, Gaudette C, Whaley F, Sauvigne A, Baribeau P, Welch HG. Telephone care as a substitute for routine clinic follow-up. JAMA 1992;267:1788–1793.

Index